RUNNING FOR OUR LIVES:

AN ODYSSEY WITH CANCER

BY
KATHRYN H. ANTHONY
WITH
BARRY D. RICCIO

Copyright© 2004 by Kathryn H. Anthony
School of Architecture
117 Temple Buell Hall
611 Taft Drive
University of Illinois at Urbana-Champaign
Champaign, IL 61820 USA
Tel: 217-244-5520
Fax: 217-244-2900
e-mail:kanthony@uiuc.edu

Printed by CPS, Facilities and Services Printing Department
54 East Gregory Drive
University of Illinois at Urbana-Champaign
Champaign, IL 61820 USA
Tel: 217-244-1455
Fax: 217-244-0414
e-mail: cps@uiuc.edu

To order more copies, contact CPS, Facilities and Services
Printing Department

Cover photographs courtesy of Rick Rickman and Kathryn H. Anthony.
Cover design by Copenhaver Cumpston.

ISBN: 0-9748450-0-0

DEDICATION

To our families and friends
To all Barry's doctors, nurses, and medical staff
To the 400 blood donors whom we will never know

In memory of my husband, hero, and best friend

TABLE OF CONTENTS

Reflections From Barry's Medical Team
(2000)

A basic biomedical scientist spends many years thinking about proteins, genes, cells, or tissues. It is rare for most of us to think about human disease unless it directly impacts us in a personal way.

Over the past ten years the research in my laboratory has taken an unexpected turn. Our basic research efforts on cancer cells and blood vessels allowed us to selectively kill tumor-associated blood vessels.

We were surprised to see how much excitement was generated by the news media over our scientific publications in this area. In fact, our publication in the journal *Cell* received international press coverage and was featured on the front page of *The New York Times*.

I had no idea what an impact this would have on my life. Based on our scientific publications and perhaps the media attention, we were able to convince a biotech company and large pharmaceutical firm to help us bring our discovery from the lab bench to the patient bedside. This took a number of years.

At this point my path crossed with Barry Riccio. Barry, who had been battling cancer for several years, learned of our discovery and the Phase I clinical trial that was being planned in San Diego. A Phase I clinical trial is typically performed on late stage cancer patients who have failed all previous treatment. It is simply designed to identify the level of toxicity as the dose of the drug is escalated. In February 1997, Barry became the second patient in the world to be treated with our drug, now named Vitaxin. As a scientist it is hard to assume that Vitaxin was responsible for Barry's improvement. Nevertheless, I do not think I could convince Barry that Vitaxin did not positively impact his disease.

During the past couple of years I have had the chance to meet Barry, his wife and mother. I began to realize our studies may have made the difference in their lives. This is when everything hit me. Over the years I had done my best to keep my professional and personal life separate. Meeting Barry and his family changed all that forever.

David A. Cheresh, Ph.D.
Professor, Departments of Immunology and Vascular Biology
The Scripps Research Institute
La Jolla, California

This is a unique history of perseverance and courage in an extraordinary fight for life conducted by an exceptionally strong individual with the constant support of family, friends, employers, and health care givers. Multiple diagnostic procedures, operations, drug treatments and transfusions as well as prolonged displacements from home would tax even the strongest of individuals. Why did so many travel the difficult road along with Barry Riccio, who has a relatively rare disease, which is generally considered hopeless? The answer lies in his infectious, enthusiastic and thoughtful appreciation not only for his own life but also that of others. After considerable research and contemplation, Barry willingly tried new, even risky, approaches because it may help others.

Serious illness unavoidably changes one's perspectives, as is evident in the pages of this book. Readers will come away knowing a remarkable individual and realize that it was and is a privilege of being one of Professor Riccio's students.

David Fromm, M.D.
Penberthy Professor and Chairman
Department of Surgery
Wayne State University
Detroit, Michigan

Why Barry Riccio developed cancer is not known, but we do know how he dealt with it. His battle with cancer is the basis for this remarkable story. We have much to learn about cancer, and stories like Barry's allow us to look back and try to uncover what allowed him to do as well as he has.

Barry benefited from two important resources. He benefited from a loving companion who was willing to battle cancer at his side. The importance of such a companion has been borne out in research showing that patients with a strong social network do better than those who are left to battle cancer "on their own."

In addition, Barry took responsibility for his own care. This was made apparent when Barry insisted on answers when answers were not given, and when he insisted on an understanding of what was being done to him. I imagine this was not always easy for him, and I know it was not easy for his medical providers. Nonetheless, through his perseverance, he reminded his care givers that we were here to serve our patients, to provide understanding, and to provide assistance in battling this terrible disease.

Certainly, a less determined person in Barry's situation would have accepted defeat much earlier and as a result, never have benefited from treatments that likely extended his life. I feel honored to have been a part of Barry's care, and I know that our understanding of cancer has been advanced as a result of his struggle.

John C. Gutheil, M. D.
Former Director, Clinical Oncology Research
Sharp HealthCare, Sidney Kimmel Cancer Center
San Diego, California

If you ever doubt what a persistent and well-motivated person with cancer can accomplish on his own behalf, spend a few hours with Barry Riccio. He will tell you that he has been lucky in the course of his cancer, but he has made his own good luck by his intense involvement in his own care. The fascinating story of this exceptional cancer patient should provide inspiration to others facing the same challenges.

Patricia A. Johnson, M.D., Ph.D.
Carle Cancer Center
Urbana, Illinois

An oncologist deals primarily with tangibles; diagnoses, dosages, measurements, and resultant therapies. But one also cannot remain unaware of the intangibles of cancer treatment; the effect of a patient's attitude; their spirit or grit, as it were. The effects of these intangible factors cannot always be denied, and I have long been interested in the role these intangible qualities may play in a patient's response to treatment.

Barry Riccio became my patient in 1997. His first cancer had been diagnosed in 1993, and he had already survived longer than had been initially anticipated. A variety of treatments and therapies had resulted in remissions, but no cures. But his attitude was confident, almost belligerent, toward his disease. He researched his diagnoses and therapies deeply and intently, and was an active participant in his treatments. Is he still alive because of this fighting spirit, and intensity of purpose? As a physician, I cannot say. But the story of his fight against his disease can only serve to inspire others, and to have been part of this fight was a lesson in the indomitability of the human spirit.

Jurgen Kogler, M.D.
Board Certified Medical Oncology
Sharp HealthCare/Scripps System
San Diego, California
Primary Investigator for Sidney Kimmel Cancer Center
La Jolla, California

As an oncology nurse, I was inspired and honored to be a part of Barry and Kathryn's life for over a year. My association with Barry began by phone as I assisted him in becoming one of the first humans to receive a phase one anti-angiogenesis monoclonal antibody.

Barry's longer-than-predicted survival is a testimony to his positive attitude and his perseverance in seeking out the newest and best of cancer treatments.

His attitude and the unending family support should be an inspiration to all cancer patients and their families proving that positive things can happen to patients—and they should never give up.

For me, the most rewarding aspect of being an oncology nurse is the satisfaction of helping patients like Barry not only live longer but also have a better quality of life.

Joy L. Hamer R.N. OCN
Former Clinical Oncology Research Nurse, Clinical Oncology Research
Sharp HealthCare, Sidney Kimmel Cancer Center
San Diego, California

ACKNOWLEDGEMENTS

Acknowledgements are due many dedicated medical staff, friends, and family who helped us through our medical odyssey.

Barry's vast medical team included numerous doctors, nurses, medical researchers, technicians, and staff. Special thanks are due Dr. David Cheresh of the Scripps Research Institute in La Jolla, California, who invented the drug, Vitaxin, that prolonged Barry's life for almost two years; as well as to Dr. Judah Folkman of Children's Hospital in Boston and Harvard Medical School, who pioneered the antiangionenesis movement that led to the development of Vitaxin.

Warm thanks are extended to numerous physicians who treated Barry with care and compassion. At Carle Hospital and Clinic in Urbana, Illinois, these included Dr. Michael Day, our longtime general practitioner; and Dr. Patricia Johnson, Barry's oncologist who provided unflagging support for over seven years. At M. D. Anderson Cancer Center in Houston, Texas, Dr. Steven Curley performed Barry's liver surgery and served as our trusted medical consultant throughout Barry's illness. At Harper Hospital in Detroit, Michigan, Dr. David Fromm performed surgery using photodynamic light therapy on Barry's greater omentum and remained in touch with us for years afterwards. At Sharp Hospital and Clinic in San Diego, surgical oncologist Dr. Robert Barone rescued Barry from a permanent gastric feeding tube; Dr. Jurgen Kogler served as Barry's steadfast oncologist for four years, skillfully handling one emergency after another; gastroenterologist Dr. Jeffrey Pressman oversaw Barry's many emergency stomach complications; and Dr. Ronald Scott performed radiation therapy on Barry's head and stomach and helped keep Barry in the Vitaxin protocol. At Sidney Kimmel Cancer Center, Drs. John Gutheil and Thomas Shiftan oversaw the Vitaxin clinical trial, advised us on numerous medical complications, and were unusually accessible to Barry. At the University of California at San Diego's Medical Center, Dr. Kenneth Binmoeller inserted the duodenal stent that allowed Barry to eat normally again.

Several nurses and medical staff routinely assisted Barry in the chemotherapy lab. We saw them so often that they became not only our medical support, but also our friends. At Carle Clinic they included Jill

Ashton, Connie Elson, Anita Lawrence, Karla Morris, Michele Perkins, Melissa Phillips, Evie Roughton, Cindy Steiger, and Janice Walker. At Sharp Infusion Therapy Center these included Diane Bradford, June Childress, Patty Felts, Kristy Fleck, Fely Fluoresca, Joy Hamer, Joan Hamrick, Adrian "A.J." Johnson, Cindy Karp, Christine Maloney, Cheryl Pettit, Lisa Prado, Mo Scarborough, and Kathy Wood. The cheerful atmosphere created in Sharp chemo lab made us actually look forward to our visits. Barry was also a regular patient at Sharp Hospital's Polinsky Oncology Unit on 8 North, where the following nurses oversaw his care: Deb Baehrenx, Massimo Breda, Haydee Dizon, Michael Drafz, Monica Fries, Angie Gonzales, Polly Guiang, Ellen Hernon, Lisa Herrera, Sheila Hershberger, Richard Skelcher, and Pat Williams.

A number of fellow cancer survivors entertained Barry—and vice versa—while undergoing chemotherapy, including Len Heumann at Carle Clinic; Connie Dorius, Bill and Adele Farr, and Stephanie Kaupp at Sharp Infusion Therapy Center.

Staff members at Island Inn bent over backwards to make us more comfortable during our San Diego stay. They included Harry Metzger, Joann Myers, Dawn Palmer, and Cris Vasquez.

Over the years, scores of friends and family visited Barry during his many hospitalizations; others delivered food or hosted us at their homes while Barry was recovering from surgery. In Urbana these included Dan and Natalie Alpert; Charlotte and Walter Arnstein; Carolyn Dry; Ralph and Ruth Fisher; Farzana and Kaizad Irani; Sharon Irish and Reed Larson; Diane LaBarbera; Casey and Mary Machula; Kathryn and Steve Marshak; Robert Ousterhout; Carole and Tino Rebeiz; Barbara and Robert Selby; Amita Sinha; Clark and Mary Lee Spence; William Sullivan; Beth Stafford-Vaughan and Ted Vaughan; Norma Vyse; and Alex and Karen Winter-Nelson. Several San Diegans extended their hospitality to us while Barry was undergoing treatment there, including Ian Abramson, Jan Bull and Ellen Kester; Bill Hargreaves; Sandy and Stephanie Kaupp; Greg and Bess Lambron; William McGill, Alex and Jeannette Rigopoulos; Daniel Shaw; and Geoffrey Wedgwood. Kris Day and Keith Woerpel offered us their cottage in Laguna Beach while

Barry was in the midst of his media blitz.

Anne and Harry Anthony, Anthony Antoniades, Felicia Riccio,Peter Pinsky, and Jack Rozos visited us while Barry was undergoing treatment at M.D. Anderson Cancer Center in Houston. Anne Anthony and Felicia Riccio accompanied us on our two visits to Harper Hospital Detroit.

Many friends and family members went out of their way to visit us—some from across the country, and some several times—while Barry was undergoing medical treatment in San Diego: Miguel Baltierra; Jami Becker; Helen and Joe Boltinghouse; Jim, Debbie, and Mollie Boltinghouse; Georgeann Burton; Eric Cammarena; Colleen Casey; Monica Chan; Dan Chin; Susan Boltinghouse-Cook and Jeff, Daniel, and Evan Cook; Lynne Curry; Robert Englund; Katie Harrison; Fred Jaher; Dean Kardassakis; Steve Kinney; Mark Kertz; Diane LaBarbera; Joanne Lagos; Herb Lasky; Minnie Loo; Casey, Mary, Hans, and Charles Machula; Sanjoy, Shampa, and Ani Mazumdar; Betsey and Craig Monsell; Yoshi Morita; Stan Nadell; Rich Nelson; Mary Nicholas; Barbara Oberto; George Peasley; Peter Pinsky; Amar Rana; Felicia Riccio; Greg, Maria, Christina and Marissa Riccio; Jack Rozos; Michael Rozos; Aphrodite Sarelas; Bruce and Beth Scheid; Eric Schmidt; Christine Self; Aileen Smith; John, Alexander, Annie, and Jeannette Smith and Mary Anne Anthony Smith; Dan, Jeanne, and Andy Stokols; Mike and Wendy Trenary; and Gary Whitmer.

Rosalie Fuentes and Richard Perry of Patient Account Services in Champaign saved us thousands of dollars in medical bills.

Colleagues who took over our classes included Terry Barnhart, Lynne Curry, Mark Leff, and Amita Sinha. Our departmental administrators Michael Andrejasich, R. Alan Forrester, and Anita Shelton provided steadfast support as well.

Several reporters covered part of Barry's medical odyssey in their news stories. They included John Crewdson of *The Chicago Tribune*; Anne Cook of the Champaign-Urbana *News Gazette*; Christine Gorman of *Time*; Vincent Kiernan of *The Chronicle of Higher Education*; Jeff Nesmith of *The Atlanta Journal-Constitution*; Leonard Novarro of the *San Diego Union-Tribune*; and E'louise Ondash of *North County Times*. Robert Cook of *Newsday* interviewed us for his book on *Dr. Folkman's War: Angiogenesis and the Struggle to Defeat Cancer* (Random House, 2001).

Lisa Busjahn, Jane Cook, Barbara Oberto, Joanna Strauss, and Amita Sinha reviewed earlier versions of this manuscript. Daniel Shaw provided key editorial advice and helped us with many medical references. Selah Peterson provided critical graphic design assistance. Cope Cumpston produced the cover design.

Numerous relatives sent Barry countless cards over the years—a collection that could fill a room. These included Antoinette Angio; Anne and Harry Anthony; Mary Jo Balacz; Stephanie Masters; Karen Mertes; Georgia Paul; George, Jon, Mary and Norah Predaris; Felicia, Gregory and Maria Riccio; Helen, Jack, Michael, and Sharon Rozos; Helen and Peter Skoufis; Mary Anne Anthony Smith and John Smith; Rob, Kris, and Kenneth Villari. Two of our adopted aunts in Chicago, Aphrodite Sarelas and Terry Ebinger, kept in constant touch with us.

Our parents, Anne and Harry Anthony, and Felicia Riccio, provided us with much-needed financial support when our funds had run dry, allowing me to take care of Barry while I was on Family and Medical Leave, as well as with moral support as we faced blow after blow. Each stood by us through thick and thin throughout our seven-year odyssey.

INTRODUCTION

During 1998 a wave of publicity about innovative approaches to treat cancer hit the newsstands. My late husband, Barry Riccio, was the beneficiary of one of these novel treatments. In these pages, I tell our story. *Running for Our Lives* is one of the first books to document the beginning of this new era in cancer research from the viewpoint of the patient, his medical team, his family, and his friends. Learning about Barry's experience empowers others to prolong their own lives and

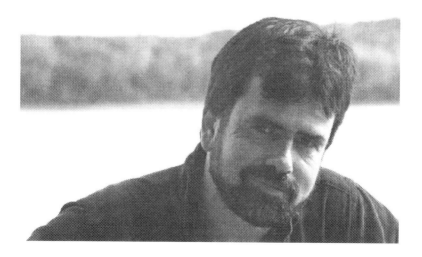

Barry a few days after learning that his cancer had spread to his liver. Brown County State Park, Indiana; October 1994. (credit: author)

the lives of those they care about. Our book is among the first to address how a patient's willingness to risk his life in a phase one clinical trial of an unknown drug changed a couple's lives dramatically. It is both a biography and an autobiography, explaining in gripping detail our seven-year emotional roller coaster ride, and especially how our research skills, our persistence, and our outreach to family and friends helped us wage our battle.

Ironically, Barry, a historian by profession, began making medical history. His quiet struggle turned public when he was thrust into the national spotlight as one of the greatest success stories in a study of desperately sick patients. In 1998 Barry's name appeared in *Time* (May 18), and he was featured in *The Chicago Tribune* (May 25), *The Chronicle of Higher Education* (May 15) and elsewhere. That same year he also appeared on ABC News with Peter Jennings (May 4) and NBC Nightly News with Tom Brokaw (May 6), whose news clips aired internationally, as well as on two nightly news broadcasts in San Diego. But each news item simply touches the tip of the iceberg. His full story needs to be told.

First diagnosed with cancer in 1993, and pronounced as terminal in 1995, Barry outlived all expectations. Even his doctors were amazed at how well he was able to stave off the inevitable. Our medical odyssey took us to several of the nation's top cancer facilities, including the Mayo Clinic in Rochester, Minnesota and MD Anderson Cancer Center in Houston, Texas. Ultimately we traveled to the noted Sidney Kimmel Cancer Center and Sharp Hospital in San Diego, California. There Barry pioneered a promising new drug which seeks to cut off cancerous tumors from their blood supply through a process called antiangiogenesis. Immunologist David Cheresh at the Scripps Research Institute in La Jolla developed the drug known as Vitaxin. Dr. Judah Folkman of Harvard University and the Children's Hospital in Boston first proposed antiangiogenesis therapy in the early 1970's, but only recently has the process been tried in humans. For well over a year, this new treatment kept his cancer at bay, and in some instances the tumors actually shrank. And for several months, even with advanced cancer throughout several organs, Barry was able to enjoy a normal life, virtually symptom free. In the 21st century, treatments like these are likely to become the wave of the future for millions around the world.

Several major themes run throughout *Running for Our Lives.*

KNOWLEDGE IS POWER

Barry would not have survived for several years with advanced, metastatic cancer had we not both conducted extensive research to learn about different treatment options. Although our local doctor was highly competent, she offered only one outside referral, which in the long run proved fruitless. All other treatments we found on our own. Both of us followed up on leads on "News from Medicine" on CNN, newspaper articles, and Web sites on the Internet. For with cancer, time is of the essence. From the onset of Barry's illness, we ordered a complete set of his medical records, allowing us to contact experts around the country on our own. We obtained not only second opinions, but also third, fourth, and fifth opinions.

THE HMO DILEMMA

Our experiences shed light on the debate over Health Maintenance Organizations (HMOs). Millions of Americans—more than half the population—are forced into HMOs, and their numbers are rising steadily. When Barry was first struck with cancer in September 1993, we were both enrolled in an HMO. We were locked into it for nine long months, but the following spring we switched to a Preferred Provider Organization. Barry changed his health plan out of necessity; I changed mine out of protest. We had both witnessed first-hand how our HMO treated us when we needed it most.

CONSULTATIONS WITH EXPERTS

Barry's physician at MD Anderson Cancer Center, Dr. Steven Curley, proved to be an invaluable resource. Although we visited him five times from 1994 to 1995, we never actually saw him after that. However, we continued to contact him intermittently to seek his advice. He availed himself whenever we needed him, steering us away from many "quack" approaches and ratifying our decisions to seek out cutting edge treatments. Likewise the many medical contacts we established across the country continued to suggest therapies that might stall Barry's cancer.

PARTICIPATION IN CLINICAL TRIALS

Statistics show that only 3-5 percent of patients with advanced cancer participate in clinical trials. Many patients simply don't know about them, as their doctors may not inform them of studies occurring outside their own medical center. Some people choose not to participate for logistical reasons, as relocating to a strange place for treatment may be impossible. Others fear the possible dire side effects described in the fine print of these protocols. Or, having already seen how chemotherapy can ravage their bodies, they prefer to die in peace. But in Barry's case, participation in a clinical trial was essential. His medical team in San Diego stressed the need for more patients to volunteer for such trials. Not only do patients stand to benefit, but also clinical trials are among the most important tools to help scientists find effective cancer treatments.

THE ROLE OF THE PHYSICAL HOUSING ENVIRONMENT

Our journey took us to a wide array of places for cancer treatment. Some were outstanding while others were woefully deficient. While Ronald McDonald houses have sprouted up throughout the US as temporary residences for cancer-ridden children and their families, few such facilities exist for adults. For people like us, finding temporary housing during treatment presented a special challenge. We spent several weeks at the Rotary House at MD Anderson Cancer Center in Houston, by far one of the nation's most state-of-the-art facilities; three long weeks at International Center/Guest Housing at the Detroit Medical Center; and in San Diego, where no such medical housing exists, we lived for over two years at Island Inn. The latter is an award-winning, federally subsidized single-room occupancy residence, both a hotel and an apartment complex. It serves as a prototype for low-to-moderate income temporary housing that is desperately needed in all major metropolitan areas across the US. For us, Island Inn was a life raft. Yet most cities have no place like it.

THE ROLE OF COLLEAGUES AND FRIENDS

But our book is more than just a story about cancer. It is a tale about two people, our relationship to each other, and our relationships with others who cared about us.

Equally important are the personal and professional contexts. Barry was an Associate Professor of History at Eastern Illinois University (EIU) in Charleston. He was the author of a book, *Walter Lippmann: Odyssey of A Liberal* (Transaction Publishers, 1994) and scores of scholarly publications. From his hospital bed, immediately after one of his operations, Barry authored a play entitled *The Review.* It was performed in January 1997 at the Charleston Alley Theatre. And even while undergoing chemotherapy, radiation, and genesis treatments, Barry continued writing his second book on American politics and society over the past quarter-century.

In April 1995, while in excruciating pain from hemorrhoids exacerbated by two and a half months of chemotherapy, Barry interviewed for a tenure-track teaching position at EIU. He had been teaching there on a full-time but temporary basis since 1991. His Sisyphean quest for a tenure-track post in his overcrowded field had lasted a decade, since receiving his doctorate in history in 1985. He was offered the permanent position at EIU in May 1995. Just a year later, in September 1996, he received tenure. His department chair, with the support of her colleagues, accelerated the review process in light of Barry's medical condition. In academic settings, where the head often trumps the heart, such actions are unheard of.

On February 12, 1997 Barry taught his final class at EIU. Late that evening, after his colleagues threw him a surprise going-away party, Barry drove out west alone, dodging snowstorms, to participate in the clinical trial. My job as a university professor forced me to stay behind. We kept in touch by our cell phone as he drove under the St. Louis Arch and across the plains of Oklahoma, the mountains of New Mexico, and the deserts of Arizona. Though we were separated for several months, we managed to spend the next two years together. The staff at my campus helped me arrange for Family and Medical Leave. Afterwards, I used up my entire sick leave, accumulated over 13 years. We temporarily gave up our comfortable nine-room house in Urbana to live in a 300 square-foot studio apartment in San Diego.

Colleagues and friends played key roles in this story. In 1995 two neighbors in Urbana informed us about photodynamic light therapy, an innovative technique used in the plant and animal world that is occasionally applied to humans. With their help we discovered a physician willing to try this procedure on Barry, even though other doctors had told us that no operation could control his cancer. At both our campuses, colleagues routinely pitched in to teach our classes when Barry was incapacitated by this illness or required to travel for medical treatment. For seven years, I have maintained an e-mail list of hundreds of "Friends of Barry," a constant source of inspiration to both of us. I have archived most of our correspondence.

———•·•———

Running for Our Lives offers an in-depth look at Barry's case, more than any news media to date have provided. Although we were unlucky in many ways, we were fortunate in the emotional and financial support we received from our employers, our family, and our friends. We realize that not everyone can do what we have done. Yet no matter what one's circumstances, our experience is instructive. When faced with adversity, we mustered whatever energy we had left, and we fought back. We refused to take "No" for an answer, to sit back and let Barry die. Somehow, from one disaster to another, we always managed to rebound. For that I have Barry to thank. While I was often on the brink of despair, he never faltered. His resilience was contagious.

More importantly, our example serves as hope and inspiration to millions of people with cancer and other serious illnesses; to their families and friends; to physicians and oncology nurses who work with cancer patients every day; to medical researchers; and to the public at large. It provides a window into our private world, one where the struggle to stay alive overshadowed all else. And it provides further impetus for all those involved in the medical community to expedite their quest for controlling—and ultimately curing—such a deadly disease.

———•·•———

I wish I could report that we were both alive and well when this book was published. But it was not meant to be. We worked on this manuscript together for several years knowing that Barry might not live to see it finished. However, he did come close. He last revised it in December 2000, and he passed away less than a month later, on January 10, 2001.

Note that most of our book is written in my voice, with Barry's voice featured in quotes and interviews. And everywhere except in this Introduction and in the Epilogue, I refer to him in the present tense. That was the way he wanted it.

Although we continued to hope for more ways to prolong his life, we both knew that Barry's resilience could not last forever. And in the end, "Bounce-Back-Barry" bounced back no more. The monster that had ravaged his body for over seven years finally won out.

During Barry's final days at San Diego's Sharp Hospital, as I watched him lying in bed, drenched in sweat, too weak to speak or even lift a cup of tea, I glimpsed out the doorway at the other cancer patients strolling in the hallways with their loved ones. How I envied them now! I flashed back to all the times when Barry had raced through those same corridors—and those in Urbana, Detroit, and Houston. A pole with a huge array of tubes and pouches dangled next to him. He sped down the hallway, pushing against his pole on wheels, his hospital gown fluttering in the breeze.

"Slow down, Barry! You're exposing yourself!" I would say to him. But I hardly had time to tie his gown before he rushed off again. And I could barely keep up with him.

"I haven't walked my mile yet!" he would say to me. "I've got to walk a mile! Exercise is good for the immune system!"

On many such occasions, I struggled to hold back tears. But in retrospect I wish I had felt differently. For after yet another close call, Barry would always come back home with me. He had won another chance at life.

In the end, we had no more chances left.

As I complete the finishing touches on *Running for Our Lives*, I can not help but wish that our story had a different ending. Is it triumph over tragedy, or tragedy over triumph? In fact, it is both. For Barry and I both believed that it is not the ending, but the journey that makes our tale unique.

As I sit in my study, staring out at our front yard on a bright, spring day, I can still see Barry charging up our walkway, carrying an armload of books. His jet-black hair is only partly obscured by his Greek fisherman's cap. His scraggly beard could use a good trim. His shirt pockets are overflowing with tiny strips of paper, candy wrappers, and receipts. His pants are wrinkled. His shoes are scuffed as usual.

Behind that rumpled façade are two deep-set, sparkling brown eyes. Amazingly, no matter how many body blows from his cancer he withstood over the years, that sparkle remained. And only in his last few hours did it begin to fade. His luminous eyes were the windows to his soul—a soul that embodied a zest for life, a desire to go on living rather than to fear dying.

As so many friends have told me, "Anyone who knew Barry will never forget him!" And although many of you may never have met him, I hope that after reading our tale, you, too, will agree.

CHAPTER ONE

Lightning Strikes Us
(1993 - 1994)

MONTAIGNE, A FRENCH WIT WHO WAS NOTED FOR HIS APHORISMS ABOUT LIFE, LOVE, AND THE HUMAN CONDITION, ONCE SAID, "HE WHO FEARS HE SHALL SUFFER ALREADY SUFFERS WHAT HE FEARS."
THERE'S AN ELEMENT OF TRUTH TO IT. I THINK WE CAN NOT HELP FEARING BUT WE CAN CERTAINLY HELP WHAT WE DO IN THE FACE OF OUR FEARS. I'VE ALMOST ALWAYS TRIED NOT TO LET MY FEARS PARALYZE ME BUT RATHER PROD ME TO ACT MORE DECISIVELY THAN I WOULD DO OTHERWISE.
—BARRY RICCIO

When I reflect upon the past seven years of our lives together, a kaleidoscope of images appears. But one stands out above all.

On Monday, September 13, 1993, lightning struck us. Our peaceful life in Urbana, Illinois, came to an abrupt end. And ever since that date things would never be the same.

That evening our good friends, Carole and Tino Rebeiz, hosted one of our neighborhood potluck parties. I arrived early. The intense heat and humidity was typical of our late Midwestern summers. Sweat was steadily dripping down my neck. With every breath I sensed the heavy, moist air. Mosquitoes were out in full force, biting me at every turn. All along the picnic tables colorful casseroles were lined up in a row. We struggled to swat the bugs away from the food.

Barry joined us later that evening after having taught his late afternoon class at Eastern Illinois University in Charleston, an hour south of Champaign-Urbana. By then the sun had already set, so I couldn't get a good look at him. I later learned that colleagues who had seen him earlier that day found him pale and wan. I had set a plate of food aside just to make sure Barry would have something to eat. He always had a reputation for a voracious appetite, he loved potluck dinners, and I didn't want him to be disappointed. He devoured his meal in seconds and chatted with several partygoers. As the party began to wind down and guests headed home, we moved into Carole and Tino's house. There we struck up a conversation with their daughter and son-in-law.

As we were saying our good-byes in the living room, Barry blurted out, "I'm not feeling very well. I need to step outside to get some air!"

Now that he was standing underneath the front porch light, I could see that his shirt and his hair were drenched in sweat. Suddenly he vomited. His head began swirling, aiming straight for the concrete. Seconds before it hit, I intercepted his fall. His Styrofoam cup slipped out of his hand and toppled onto the steps.

Seconds later Barry came back to life. Carole offered him a fresh glass of water and escorted him back into the family room. I remember watching Barry's soiled shirtsleeve grazing ever so slightly against the couch. We made an SOS call to our neighbor, Brad Katz, a medical student who had been at the party earlier that evening with his wife and son. Brad arrived instantly. With just one look, he could see that Barry was extremely pale. He took Barry's pulse and found it weak.

Once Barry regained his strength, Tino and I each wrapped an arm around his shoulders. The three of us slowly walked down the front steps, turned left onto the sidewalk, past the two houses in between us, and left again onto our front walk.

"Get yourself to a doctor tomorrow," Tino warned us. "You need a thorough physical examination. You never know what this could be."

Once Tino left, I helped Barry onto our living room couch to lie down. As he rested, I drew the bath water upstairs, hoping that it would refresh him. Yet even after his bath, as he settled back onto the couch, I noticed that he was still white as snow. He was glassy-eyed and weak. His toenails and fingernails had no color at all. I phoned the Patient

Advisory Nurse at Carle Hospital and described Barry's symptoms.

"Keep an eye on him and call us back again soon," she said.

After my second call about an hour later, I put Barry on the line.

The nurse said to him, "It could simply be heat exhaustion, but it could be much more serious. Staying home could be dangerous. It's best that you come in and be evaluated."

So at about 11:30 p.m., we sped off to the Emergency Room. I left the outside light on, just in case I had to return home alone.

By 2 a.m. Barry was lying on a gurney, dressed in a hospital gown. He was being examined by one of the emergency room physicians, a somewhat brusque fellow.

"It sure looks like a bleeding ulcer to me," the doctor stated.

Nurses soon hooked Barry onto an intravenous tube, pricking and poking as they searched for his vein.

The doctor asked me, "Do you authorize us to do a blood transfusion? His hemoglobin level is only 6.3. That's dangerously low. You know the hazards. But at this point you really have no choice."

"Go ahead," I said.

Within seconds someone else's blood began dripping out of the plastic pack. I was awestruck. It was a sight I had never seen before.

At the same time, the doctor began cramming a nasogastric tube through Barry's nose and down his throat.

I tried to make it easier by joking with Barry, "Don't worry. Just pretend you're delving into some delicious pasta!"

Barry was not amused. As he struggled to swallow the tube, he winced and gasped for breath. Never had I seen Barry look so frightened. Soon he was enveloped by a maze of tubes, packs, and poles. In just a few minutes he had been transformed from person to patient. It was a change I would witness several times over.

"It sure looks like a bleeding ulcer to me," said the doctor.

Hours later transporters sped Barry through a maze of hallways, up the elevator, through yet another maze of corridors, past a nursing station, and up to his hospital room. I dashed to keep up with the entourage, who seemed to have forgotten my existence. With no chance to catch my breath and look around, I had no idea where I was going.

After helping Barry settle into his room, I could see that the commotion had taken its toll. His eyelids started to droop, his voice dimmed, and he began to doze. I realized that it was time for me to go home. Oddly enough, although it was way past my usual bedtime, I wasn't even tired. Ever since the incident on our neighbors' front steps, my adrenaline had been pumping away at full force.

As I left Barry's room at 5:30 a.m., I glanced at a sign above the hallway. It said "Oncology." Although I was familiar with many medical terms, this was one I did not recognize.

"Never mind," I thought. "I'll find out tomorrow."

I navigated through the maze to the elevator, a deserted corridor and finally outside. I ended up in an alley that was pitch dark.

Soon I began to panic. By now it dawned on me that I was a ripe target for a crime. I was distraught, I was alone, and I was carrying two wallets full of money—along with a real give-away: a large plastic bag labeled "Patient's Belongings." Plus I was lost.

Finally, way off in the distant parking lot, I spotted my car. It seemed like days since I had last seen it. At that moment, I felt as if I had found a long-lost friend.

Although I was still shaky, I gripped the steering wheel and drove home. Just as the sun was rising at about 6:00, I tucked myself into bed. By then the all-night trauma of the Emergency Room had left me both wired and tired.

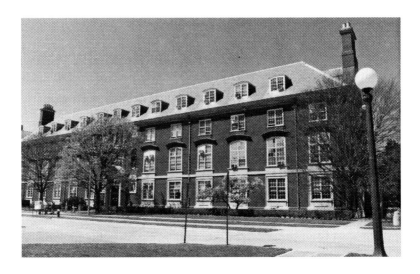

The Architecture Building at the University of Illinois at Urbana-Champaign. My office is the second dormer from the right. Champaign, Illinois; April 1999. (credit: author)

On Tuesday morning I woke up around 10:00. An hour later I was on the University of Illinois campus sitting in a circle with my colleagues at a design faculty meeting. I felt as if I were in a daze, and I could barely keep my eyes open.

At about 3:00 p.m. I called the hospital to check up on Barry.

A nurse answered, "Mr. Riccio? He's been moved to the Intensive Care Unit."

"What for?"

"He's having a series of tests. Call me when you get here and I'll take you to him."

As I hung up the phone, my adrenaline surged once more. I dashed out the door and sped down the elevator. My only detour was to the departmental office.

"Barry's in the hospital. He's taken a turn for the worse. I may not be back for a while," I told the secretaries.

Little did I know then that I would not return to school for almost two weeks.

Outside I could see a fierce wind blowing and black clouds threatening overhead. I recognized that sight all too often this time of year, and it filled me with a sense of impending doom. As I sprinted through the parking lot, I was in the midst of a torrential downpour. Lightning bolts filled the sky, and thunder shook the ground. Not having checked the weather forecast, I had no raincoat, no windbreaker, and no umbrella. By the time I reached my car, my feet were soaked.

———•+•———

The hospital garage was packed. Once again I plowed through the thundershower. I called the nurse who had spoken to me over the phone. She escorted me to a yellow room marked "Endoscopy," another medical term I had never heard before.

There I met Dr. Joel Lans, a gastroenterologist. He had just finished performing an endoscopy on Barry and was reviewing the results with Dr. Lyn Tangen, a surgeon. I soon learned that an endoscopy was a test allowing doctors to view the inside of the stomach. Patients are given a strong anesthetic that prevents them from remembering the procedure. A video camera is inserted through the throat, down the esophagus and into the stomach, and a set of still images is taken. In the meantime I found Barry lying on a gurney, still groggy from the drugs.

Dr. Lans told me, "I found a tumor in Barry's stomach. But it is probably benign. Don't worry."

"We'll have to operate tomorrow," Dr. Tangen said.

Even the word "tumor" was unfamiliar to me. I flashed back to fourth grade when my best friend's dog had a tumor and died. But since then I hadn't given the word a second thought.

Shortly afterwards, transporters zoomed Barry into his room in the Intensive Care Unit (ICU). The scene made my stomach begin to churn. In one ICU waiting room, two people were sprawled out on a couch, their clothing strewn all over the floor. Others were watching TV with glazed looks in their eyes. Another group was huddled together crying. A series of signs cautioned visitors. "Only family members allowed." "Only one or two visitors at a time." Although Barry's was a large, private room, he was too sick to enjoy it. It was filled with an assortment of computer screens and monitors measuring blood pressure, heartbeat and other vital signs. Every few seconds the machines emitted strange beeps. Nearby was a jumble of poles hooked up to dripping packs of blood and clear liquids. To add to the confusion, a steady stream of nurses, orderlies, and lab technicians paraded in and out of the room.

After spending the rest of the evening at the hospital with Barry, I headed home. I called my research assistant to ask for help with my classes, and to put a note on my office door explaining my absence. Throughout Barry's hospital stay, we kept in touch daily via voice mail. Later that evening, she and her roommate sent Barry a gorgeous bouquet of flowers. Knowing that they were both starving students, I was deeply touched.

I spoke with Barry's doctor that night and learned that his condition was still very grave. Despite the many blood transfusions he had already received, his red blood count, or hemoglobin was still low. If it didn't rise significantly—to 10 at least—he might not be able to withstand an operation. Or he could bleed to death overnight. I remember lying in bed that night, tossing and turning, praying, "Please don't take him away from me!" I hardly slept at all.

I arrived back at the hospital early Wednesday morning. I carried in my own version of a bouquet, a large cardboard cutout photo of a dozen red roses sitting in a glass vase. On the back it said, "Never needs watering." I thought it might liven up Barry's spirits, but he was too sick to notice. I also brought him a favorite photo of the two of us taken at a taverna in Greece where we had visited a few summers ago. It had lived on our refrigerator door for years. I hoped it would remind us both of more pleasant times. Along with the photo was a get well card telling Barry how much I loved him. Remembering what the doctor had told me the night before, I didn't want Barry to go into surgery with any unfinished business of mine left behind.

Barry's operation was scheduled for mid-morning. Transporters came to take him away around noon. But after waiting in the pre-operating area for several hours, we were informed of a scheduling problem. Transporters then wheeled him back to his room in the ICU. By this time our friend and former next door neighbor, Norma Vyse, had stopped by for a visit. Despite the dire circumstances, all three of us managed to laugh, struck by the surreal nature of the hospital scene.

By early evening, Barry's operation finally took place. Shortly afterwards, Norma returned to keep me company in the surgical waiting area, although she soon left for a dinner appointment. She volunteered to return afterwards, so I asked if she could sneak me in a doggie bag from the restaurant. Although I was already feeling hunger pangs, I knew that I couldn't leave the scene. So a few hours later while Barry was still in surgery, I disobeyed the "No Food or Drink Allowed" signs and dove into a delicious pasta dinner. I was rejuvenated.

A hospital volunteer sat next to the phone. Whenever it rang, she shouted out, "Will the family of (patient's name) please come to the desk? The doctor wants to speak with you."

Within seconds, one or two worn-out people dragged themselves out of their seats. Shortly after, a doctor appeared to meet with them. Most of these conversations took place in the waiting room, and I could hear almost everything they were saying. After what seemed like an eternity, Barry's name was called. I darted over to the desk.

"Are you Mrs. Riccio?" the volunteer asked.

"Yes, I am."

I was too exhausted to inform her that we had different last names.

"The surgeon, Dr. Tangen, is ready to meet with you."

When the doctor arrived, he pointed towards a tiny room off the waiting area. "Let's meet in here," he suggested.

"Why are we meeting in a separate room?" I wondered. "Why can't we meet in the waiting area, just like everyone else?"

A sick feeling in my stomach warned me that something had gone awry. Norma joined me as we closed the door behind us.

Dr. Tangen explained, "The operation was a success. We were able to remove the entire tumor in the stomach muscle lining."

That was good news. He drew a diagram to show us exactly where the problem was located.

"It was at the edge of the pancreas, but luckily it had not invaded it. Had we not caught it in time, it probably would have, and this would be very, very serious. The tumor was exceptionally large: 12 centimeters. It's the size of a grapefruit!

"Based on my experience, right now I'd narrow down my diagnosis to one of three possibilities: 1) a benign tumor called leiomyoma; 2) lymphoma; or 3) leiomyosarcoma. The latter two are cancerous. Only after the pathologist examines the tumor in detail will we know for sure. You'll have to wait another few days, Friday at the earliest."

I felt like a bolt of lightning shot right through me. Never had I even suspected cancer. Barry had seemed so healthy. And he hadn't had any warning signs at all.

"How could something this serious surface so suddenly? It's incredible!" I thought.

Although my hands were shaking and my eyes were filling up with tears, I feverishly began taking notes. It was the start of my account of Barry's medical condition, one that would soon mushroom into several filing cabinets. Days later I recounted the episode over the phone to my Uncle Peter in Washington, DC.

"Whenever you get bad news," he said, "Take notes. That way you can concentrate on what the doctor is saying."

It was a useful lesson.

About an hour later Barry was released from the recovery room, his sheets and hospital gown still splattered with blood. He was as white as a sheet as he whispered to me, "I'm in so much pain!"

That dreadful image will remain with me as long as I live.

When I returned home late that night, I looked up the three medical scenarios that Dr. Tangen had described in two of my hefty medical reference books. Much to my surprise, none of those terms was even listed.

"He's so bad off that what he has can't even be found in the medical books!" I said to myself.

That Thursday Barry was moved from the ICU to a surgical recovery wing. I was disappointed that his new room was about half the size of his previous one, and even worse, he had a roommate. But that turned out to be a blessing in disguise. For the roommate was about to be released the next day, and he and his friends were in the midst of a Rosh Hashanah celebration. They were a jovial bunch. Their laughing and singing cast a festive mood on our ominous circumstances.

Once I realized that the other half of the room would soon be vacated, I headed to the nurse's station.

"When his roommate checks out tomorrow, can Barry have the window seat?" I asked.

"We prefer not to change a patient's location unless medically necessary. But here is the name of the head nurse. Why don't you ask her?"

I did, this time citing some research by one of my colleagues, Roger Ulrich, at Texas A & M University, that had been published in *Science* magazine years ago. I often referred to Roger's medical research in my classes. His studies demonstrated that hospital patients with a view of nature recovered more rapidly from surgery than those who faced a brick wall.

"Having a view helps patients recover faster," I argued. "Can't you please move him to the window?"

This was enough to convince the head nurse that I knew what I was talking about, so she agreed. The next day Barry had a room with a view.

That afternoon our neighbor, Brad and his family stopped by. I was especially happy to see them as they had been with us the night when Barry collapsed. And I felt reassured to have a friend who knew much more than I did about medicine.

"Everyone needs a few friends who are doctors," I thought to myself.

On Friday I returned to the hospital. Barry and I anxiously awaited news from the pathologist, Dr. Wellman. Oddly enough, we had actually met him and his wife earlier that summer. A former student of mine, Kaizad, had designed some new landscaping and a small pond in Dr. Wellman's backyard, and he had suggested we stop by to see it. Kaizad was helping us redesign our own front yard, and while Barry was hospitalized, we were in the midst of a major construction project at home.

Later that day, I phoned Dr. Wellman at the hospital's pathology lab and reminded him of our meeting a few months ago.

"I probably won't have the results until after the weekend, but from what I can see so far, it looks like what I suspected," he told me.

However, he didn't reveal what that was.

"We are both anxious to learn the results," I explained. "If there is any way you could let us know before then, I would appreciate it."

By now the suspense was beginning to haunt us.

Late that afternoon, our friend, Amita, stopped by for a visit with a bouquet of flowers. She was wearing one of her colorful saris. She, too, had just learned of Barry's emergency hospitalization and offered to help out with my courses. Amita and I had studied under the same faculty at Berkeley, and she knew the material, so I gladly took her up on her offer. She substituted for my seminar several times during my absence. It took a tremendous load off my mind. While immersed in our conversation, Dr. Wellman walked in.

"Should I step outside?" Amita asked.

"Only if you want to," I replied. "We don't mind if you stay."

So she remained. We introduced her to Dr. Wellman.

He then proceeded to tell us, "I've just completed the tests, and knew that you were anxious to hear the results before the weekend. They confirmed my suspicions: the tumor removed from Barry's stomach muscle lining is leiomyosarcoma. It's cancerous."

All three of us were in shock. Barry sat up straight and braced himself against the headboard. His eyes widened as he glared directly at the doctor.

"Cancer! You're not saying I have cancer, are you?" he asked. His voice was more spirited than usual, and I could read the fear in his face.

"Yes, I am," said the doctor.

Placing her hand on her head, Amita turned away and looked at the wall. I couldn't believe my ears, and I could feel my heart racing.

"It can't be true! Not Barry! He's only 38." I thought to myself. "We're both too young for this. Not now!"

But aloud I said nothing. Instead I rushed over to Barry's bedside and held his hand. Then we began asking several questions.

"Of the three scenarios, leiomyoma, lymphoma, and leiomyosarcoma, which one is the worst?"

"Actually leiomyoma would have been the best. That's a benign tumor, not a cancer. And lymphoma would be even worse. But the problem with leiomyosarcoma is that it's extremely rare. In fact, in the past eight years, I've only seen two such cases here in Champaign-Urbana."

Soon afterwards, Dr. Wellman disappeared. The three of us were left reeling from the news.

Shortly after Amita left, Ruth appeared. A nurse at the hospital, she is the wife of an architecture colleague. It was the first time I had seen Ruth on the job.

"I heard you were in here," she said, "And I wanted to come and see how you were doing."

She greeted each of us with a warm hug. In the midst of the vast medical maze, finding a friend who knew the ropes was reassuring.

Now I also began to realize, "Not only is it good to have friends who are doctors. It's good to have friends who are nurses!"

We informed Ruth about the diagnosis. She responded calmly.

"Oh, I see. Well, at least now you know what it is. That's good."

I thought to myself, "She's probably seen everything, so nothing surprises her. I wish I could sound as composed as she is about all this."

Later that day, two other friends stopped by who had been at our neighborhood block party on that fateful night. We shared the diagnosis with them. It felt strange just to say the words "cancer" and "Barry" in the same sentence. I could tell from the looks in their eyes that they were in shock.

On Friday night my parents phoned from California. When I informed them of Barry's diagnosis, all I heard on the other end of the phone was an eerie silence. Neither of them had ever suspected that Barry could have been so sick.

I soon learned that bad news spreads like wildfire. During the next several days whenever I was home from the hospital my phone wouldn't stop ringing. Every time I sat down to eat, open my mail, or pay a bill, all I heard was "ring, ring, ring." Although I appreciated everyone's concern, the steady stream of calls wore me out. I felt like a broken record, repeating the same story over and over again. I wished I could just put our tale of woe on a machine and press "play" whenever the phone rang. By the time I finally went to bed each night it was well past midnight. One night, with an ice-cold dinner still in front of me, I was still talking on the phone at 1 a.m. Early the next morning, another set of phone calls woke me up. It was overwhelming.

But in the hospital it was different. As more and more friends learned about our plight, Barry had more and more visitors. We both welcomed them with open arms. And as Barry regained his strength, I soon steered many phone calls directly to him. Despite the fact that he was still entangled in an array of tubes, especially the nasogastric tube that made it uncomfortable for him to speak, he didn't mind talking on the phone. In fact, he loved it.

Within a few days I mailed away a handful of SOS postcards to some of our closest friends who lived far away. I sent one off to Oregon and a few others to California. All I could think was that with cancer you have to move as fast as you can. So I didn't want to waste any time. The postcards showed a threatening, dark gray sky, the kind often accompanied by a tornado warning. That image couldn't have captured our mood any better. On each card I wrote a brief message:

"Barry collapsed and fainted at a party on September 13. He has been in the hospital ever since. He had an operation that revealed that he has cancer. If you'd like to call him at the hospital, I'm sure he'd be happy to hear from you. His number is...."

As soon as our friends received the postcards, they all called right back. Barry was energized by all the calls. More flowers began to fill the room. At one point I even brought in my garden clippers from home so that I could take care of all the plants.

Soon we had to choose an oncologist. After reviewing a list of names, we selected Dr. Patricia Johnson. I had heard good things about her from one of my colleagues, whose husband died of cancer years ago. Plus by that time the medical environment and its apparent sexism already disheartened me. Just about every doctor we had seen so far was a man, while just about every nurse we had seen was a woman. The fact that Dr. Johnson defied this stereotype was a point in her favor, at least as far as I was concerned.

When Barry first met Dr. Johnson, he was speed walking up and down the corridor, a habit that served him well in this and subsequent hospital stays. Dr. Johnson joined him as they walked and talked their way down the hallway. She may have found Barry amusing, as she was accustomed to speaking with patients either in her office or in their hospital beds.

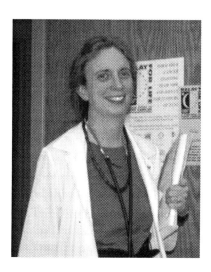

Dr. Patricia Johnson of the Carle Cancer Clinic was Barry's oncologist since his illness was first diagnosed. Urbana, Illinois; April 1999. (credit: author)

When Barry asked Dr. Johnson about the outlook for someone with leiomyosarcoma, she replied, "Well, it's certainly not dismal."

But she stressed that because her primary experience was in breast cancer, and because none of the Carle staff specialized in Barry's illness, we needed to consult with yet another physician—an expert from a major cancer center—regarding Barry's treatment. She mentioned that Carle had a connection with the Mayo Clinic in Rochester, Minnesota.

We asked to have a sample of Barry's tumor slides sent to Mayo for further analysis. After a few weeks, Mayo clinicians confirmed the original diagnosis. And in order to pursue further medical advice, we needed to go out of town—and we had no time to spare. For the first time, we recognized the drawbacks of living in a small college town. If one is in fine health, Champaign-Urbana is a great place to be. But if one has an obscure ailment, it is not. We were forced to take matters into our own hands.

With that in mind, in the first of several desperate attempts to learn more about Barry's disease, I began reading up on leiomyosarcoma. I started in the Carle Hospital library while Barry was still lying in his bed upstairs. By the time he was released I had visited that library several times.

Early in my search, I came across an article written by a Mayo Clinic physcian describing leiomyosarcoma patients and their survival rates. I learned that by the time five years were up, hardly any patients were still alive. My eyes welled up with tears as I studied one graph after another. Barry couldn't even bring himself to finish the article. I discovered several research publications about leiomyosarcoma, including one by Dr. Raphael Pollock of the MD Anderson Cancer Center in Houston, Texas. The picture Pollock painted was not a pretty one. I copied as many articles as I could find, read them at home, and filed them away in what had now become Barry's cancer file.

Like a detective, I began tracking down doctors around the country, who authored the pieces I had just read. I even called a doctor I had seen on CNN's "News from Medicine." While most people I reached were eager to help, the person who answered at the famed Sloan Kettering Cancer Center in New York City was all too brusque.

"Our doctors only speak with current patients," she said. "If you need any more information, you have to travel to New York City to meet with the doctors in person. Otherwise we can't help you."

That instantly ruled out Sloan Kettering. Facing cancer was stressful enough, but the prospect of battling it out in New York City—with surly staff like her—was just too much.

A few doctors asked for reports from Barry's recent surgery. We soon realized the value of having all his medical records in our hands. In short order we got in the habit of asking for a copy of all his medical records—and especially the reports from the surgeon and the pathologist. This way we were able to fax information directly—bypassing layers of bureaucratic red tape along the way—to whoever might be able to help us.

In the meantime, friends from both Champaign-Urbana and Charleston continued to visit Barry in the hospital every day. He was gradually regaining his energy, and the company brightened our spirits. Calls continued to pour in from far and wide. Get well cards arrived in our mailbox daily. Friends rallied to my rescue at home as well. When I returned late one night, I opened our front door to get our mail. Much to my surprise, I discovered a care package along with a delicious pot of borscht from our friends, Casey and Mary. Casey had been one of Barry's graduate students, and Mary was a nurse.

Over the phone Mary advised me, "Don't assume the doctors will tell you all you need to know. You have to do much of the work yourself. You need to be a patient advocate for Barry." It was the first I had heard this term, but I would hear it again often. Her advice made a strong impression on me.

Friends delivered bags full of groceries to my doorstep. I had neither the time nor the energy to even set foot in a grocery store. My gas tank was literally running on empty. The outpouring of affection was phenomenal. And in this respect, our small college town was incredibly supportive, and I couldn't imagine a better place to be.

Soon after Barry entered the hospital, I needed to contact his family. His mother, Felicia, and brother, Greg, lived in Arizona. But Felicia was on one of her many international tours, this time in Eastern Europe. Reaching her was not easy. I first called Greg and his wife, Maria, to break the news. In the meantime I tracked down Felicia's travel agent, who gave me the name of the tour guide and a few hotels and cities where they were likely to be that day. I called Europe late at night to see if I could reach her early the next morning. First I tried Eastern Germany, only to learn that Felicia's tour group had already come and gone. After a few more near misses, I tracked down the tour guide in Warsaw, Poland. I recounted our tale and asked for advice on how to handle Barry's mother, then 77 years old and in a fragile emotional state.

The guide explained, "I have lots of experience delivering bad news. This is an unpleasant but necessary part of my job. The best way is for me to tell Felicia myself. That would give her a chance to absorb the news first-hand before speaking with you. Why don't you give me her son's phone number in the hospital and she can call him directly?"

The next day Felicia reached Barry. She was in a panic.

"I'll cut my trip short and fly straight to Illinois," she said.

But Barry advised against this.

"Stick with your original travel plans," he said, "and come see us when you're back in the US."

So Felicia completed her Eastern European tour, flew to Chicago, and landed in Urbana near the end of Barry's hospital stay. When I picked her up from the airport, I was wiped out. And I could almost hear my stomach churning.

"Barry is in the hospital with cancer, and now his mother is going to see him for the first time. I feel like I'm in a soap opera," I thought to myself.

During my short drive with Felicia to Carle Hospital, in an attempt to defuse the tension, I played a tape by one of my favorite jazz artists. "Linus and Lucy," the theme from *A Charlie Brown Christmas* didn't really fit the occasion, but at least it was upbeat. And I thought it might help keep my blood pressure down. Hours before I had consulted with the hospital staff to help orchestrate Felicia's arrival.

"She has a history of manic depression," I had explained. "And this might just be too much for her. I'm worried that she may become hysterical—or even collapse."

"Well then, why don't you have Barry meet her in the waiting room?" one of the nurses suggested. "He can sit in a chair and appear more normal than he would lying in his hospital bed. We often think it's a good idea—if it's physically possible—when a relative sees a patient for the first time. It calms them down."

Barry and I agreed. As soon as his mother and I entered the lobby of the hospital, I called his room. When we exited the elevator, we found Barry walking to the waiting room. Just as the nurse predicted, Felicia was surprised to see him looking so good. By this time his color had returned, and for nearly a week, he had been walking the hospital corridors at least three miles a day. Felicia stayed at our house for another few weeks while I went back to work. Altogether Barry missed five weeks of teaching—one-third of the semester. On both his campus and mine, several colleagues took over our classes. It was one of the biggest favors they could do for us.

When I first returned to the School of Architecture, I felt like Rip Van Winkle. Even though it had only been two weeks since I was last on campus, it seemed like years. I had spent so many hours at the Carle Hospital that I began to feel as if I worked there. Carrying my sack lunch in the morning, I waited along with the nurses, technicians, and orderlies for the employee shuttle van. A security escort drove me back to my car later that night. The sterility of the medical environment made a strong impression on me. I dreaded the stark, institutional corridors, especially the claustrophobic, underground passage connecting the hospital and clinic. I despised the crowded waiting rooms with their blaring TVs. And I hated the antiseptic patient rooms; with just one step into the doorway, I got a whiff of that hospital stench. I could hardly stomach it.

And, after all this, I saw the university with a fresh set of lenses. The students seemed younger, happier and healthier. The campus buildings appeared grander, more stately than before, like architectural monuments. What had been mere groves of trees before now looked like forests to me. Even the Quad now took on the air of a national park.

"How fortunate I am to work in a setting as lovely as this—instead of a hospital!," I thought to myself. "I'll never take it for granted again."

I also came to view my field from a different perspective, one that stuck with me ever since. No longer did I believe architecture to be simply another profession, like medicine and law. It dawned on me that clients usually turn to architects because something good is happening. They are growing, changing, reorganizing, and entering a new phase. A family has acquired enough money to build a new house, an institution is ready to establish a new identity, or a company seeks to present a new image to the public. Compared to so many other lines of work, architecture is unusually upbeat. Never before had I been so philosophical about my profession.

All the while, our friends continued to do whatever they could for us. Now I could see why the Midwest was known as the Heartland. One friend, who didn't even own a car and lived across town volunteered to help us with yard work. Others delivered homemade lasagna, minestrone soup, and zucchini bread. Still others adorned our house with countless bouquets of flowers. And our neighbor, Carole, drove Felicia to mass on Sundays. She and Tino invited us to their home for dinner many times.

Two other neighbors, Natalie and Dan brought over tasty casseroles, one day after another. Natalie took Felicia out to lunch. Over the years she would make a habit of treating my mother-in-law whenever she came to town. Natalie cooked for us countless times. Even today, I can still hear her voice on our answering machine.

"Hello, Kathy and Barry. This is Natalie calling. We'd like to invite you over for Sunday supper."

Whether it was her famous squash soup, or chicken with red pepper jelly sauce, her gourmet dinners were better than any restaurant in town. Their living room soon became like a second home to us.

Although they were well into their 70's, this couple led an active life and traveled far and wide. A workaholic by day, Dan was an athlete by night. He worked out regularly and did aerobics at the local gym for an hour and a half each time. He often referred to his exercise as "a positive addiction." It was a phrase that would eventually rub off on me. Little did we know it at the time, but Natalie was suffering from a serious heart condition. When she died suddenly three years later, it was as if I had lost a family member. I couldn't bear to look at their house out my window, knowing that she would never return. And for a while the roles were reversed, as I delivered casseroles to Dan's front door.

Later, another friend, Rich, would become a similar role model for me. Rich had lost his young daughter to cancer. During her long illness, he took up running, and he has been an athlete ever since.

"Exercise helped me deal with stress more than just about anything else," he told me.

On September 28, after two and a half weeks in captivity, Barry was finally released from the hospital. When we pulled up our driveway, he could see that the house looked different. Our new front deck, trellis, and landscaping were now almost finished, and our yard had been transformed into a Garden of Eden. Over the next few weeks, several friends visited us at home, and we entertained them on our new deck. Barry rested and caught up on his reading and class preparation. He and Carole took several walks around our neighborhood. He especially enjoyed the tranquillity of Carle Park, only two blocks away. Between the park and our new deck, he spent much of his time outdoors enjoying the fall foliage. Our two huge maple trees turned bright yellow and were at their peak for about two weeks.

During his hospital stint Barry dropped 22 pounds, as throughout most of his stay there his diet had been reduced to sucking on ice chips. This was a special hardship for Barry, who loved to eat. As he can attest,

> When I was a junior in high school, my first month in
> Arizona, I worked at a concession stand for the football games
> at Peoria High School. I sold hot dogs, candy bars, and Cokes.
> One of the fringe benefits of the job was that I was allowed to
> eat unlimited food. And typically, I used to have four hot dogs
> and about five candy bars. But after I was working there for

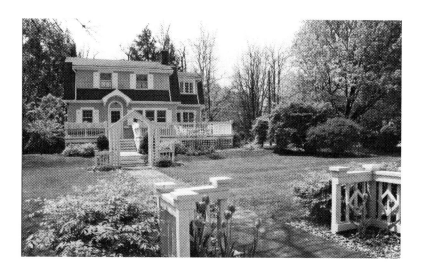

Even on our darkest days, our cheerful Dutch Colonial house brightened our spirits. Urbana, Illinois; April 1994. (credit: author)

about three weeks, Mr. Ligget, my chemistry teacher who was in charge of the concession, changed the policy. Now we were allowed only one of each. I thought it might have been because of me. In those days I really had a bottomless pit.

My senior year in high school, I worked at Sir George's Royal Buffet in Sun City. I was a busboy. There too, the best part of working there was that I was allowed all the food I wanted, although I had to pay $1 for lemonade or iced tea. So typically I had two helpings of four entrees each, and then a number of side dishes too, not to mention appetizers and dessert. There was ham with raisin pineapple sauce—one of my favorites, nice and sweet, often a fried chicken dish, casserole, and pasta. I was hungry, and at that point in my life I didn't have an especially discriminating palate. I must have had a very fast metabolism, because I wasn't skinny, but I wasn't overweight. At just under 5'11", I weighed about 150 lbs.

Over the years, his taste buds improved, and in Champaign-Urbana, Barry had become known as an amateur gourmet chef. While he relied on recipes early on in our marriage, and our cookbook collection mushroomed to over 100, he soon graduated to a higher level. Whenever he had an urge to whip up something special, he would study several recipes, close the books, and let his imagination run wild. At one point I finally forced him to dictate his recipes to me.

"After all, Barry, you might get run over by a truck someday," I prodded him.

We collected some of his recipes and distributed them to friends in a two-volume cookbook entitled *The Best of Barry.* Among the more notable meals were his own concoction of stuffed shells: a blend of the traditional tomato, onion, garlic, oregano, red wine, along with a Eurasian twist of citronella, coconut curry powder, soy sauce, and ginger. The famous novelist, Saul Bellow, had inspired that particular recipe. Barry's Southwestern pasta sauce featured prickly pear jelly, hot jalapeño honey mustard, pureed red peppers, green pepper jelly, cinnamon, cloves, cumin, hot New Mexican chili powder, Santa Fe pesto, and cactus salsa. For friends and family alike, and especially for me, tasting Barry's exotic dishes was always a special treat.

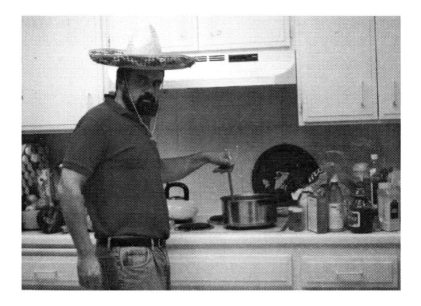

Among friends and family alike, Barry has long had a reputation as a gourmet chef. Here he is whipping up a Southwestern style meatball dish. Irvine, California; December 1990. (credit: Mary Anne Anthony Smith)

In mid-October I left for a brief speaking engagement to the University of Minnesota at Duluth. It was the first time I left Barry after he had been diagnosed with cancer. After that, I made only a handful of business trips. I was reluctant to travel far away as I had in the past, fearing that if something happened to me, Barry would have to face his illness alone. Nevertheless, he always encouraged me to go.

Barry returned to work in mid-October. And for a while, life felt almost back to normal. We took our annual fall foliage tour of Brown County State Park and Monroe Reservoir in Indiana. The blazing red, orange and yellow leaves looked as if they had leapt out of a postcard. It was one of those magical Midwestern scenes. But despite the sunshine and the fresh country air, I couldn't stop thinking about Barry's illness.

"What if he doesn't make it to his 39th birthday?" I wondered. "How many visits to Brown County will we have left together? Could this be our last one?"

Questions like these would continue to eat away at me. No matter how hard I tried to shut them out of my mind, they always seemed to rise to the surface.

After hiking around the park, we devoured a delicious apple crisp made with Jonathan apples, brown sugar and cinnamon. Barry has a special affection for cinnamon. In fact, as a small child, his family sometimes called him "the cinnamon kid."

By that time our new deck and landscaping were also complete. We had two new lilac trees, two serviceberry trees, a dogwood, a row of mission arborvitae, as well as a redbud and several batches of mums that were all in bloom. I had watered them daily and enjoyed watching all our new vegetation take off. The finishing touch was installing the lighting in and around the deck and trellis. The first night we lit up our yard I was ecstatic. We couldn't believe that this stunning spectacle was actually ours. The reincarnation of our house served as a beacon of hope.

——•◆•——

We continued to meet with Dr. Johnson that fall. She reiterated that Barry required treatment from a major cancer center, and she referred us to the Mayo Clinic in Minnesota. At the same time, she warned us that our Health Maintenance Organization (HMO) would not pay for any consultation there. I called Mayo and learned that it cost $1500 simply to walk in the door. We traveled to Minnesota in November 1993.

Our visit to the Mayo Clinic required that we once again take time off from work. I regretted being away just on the heels of my absence two months earlier, but I had little choice. The drive to Minnesota took eight long hours.

As we approached Rochester from the freeway, we could see the skyline off in the distance. Although ominous clouds loomed overhead, the sun was shining on a jumble of tall buildings comprising the Mayo Clinic and St. Mary's Hospital. From afar it looked like the Land of Oz. Could this be our medical Mecca? We could only hope so.

We arrived at about 4:30 Wednesday afternoon, just in time to hand-deliver Barry's latest CT-scans, chest X-rays, and medical records to the doctors. It had taken us several days to collect them all from Carle Hospital before we left Urbana. We had guarded them in the back seat of our car during our long ride.

Thursday morning when we checked in for our appointment, the doctor told us that he could not locate any information about Barry. His staff's search for Barry's scans revealed nothing at all. We were both outraged.

"Fifteen hundred dollars and our records are lost overnight, just like that. What kind of place is this, anyway?" we asked ourselves.

We insisted on not leaving the clinic until our documents were found. Needless to say, it did not make a good first impression.

By Friday our records were magically discovered. We were then sent to three different doctors who advised us on what to do next. The first suggested external radiation aimed at the abdomen. The second recommended intra-operative radiation therapy, a technique whereby Barry's stomach would be surgically opened up and radiation would be applied. This could take place over Christmas at their own St. Mary's Hospital. Needless to say, it didn't sound like the best way to spend the upcoming holiday season. The third physician, an expert on leiomyosarcoma and the one whose articles we had read, had yet a different point of view. Unlike the previous two physicians, he believed that radiation might be harmful to the abdomen. But more importantly, he stressed that it was pointless to radiate one part of the body when, because of the systemic nature of the illness, the cancer could easily spread elsewhere. He thought that Barry would be better off merely having the cancer monitored approximately once every three months. Finally, before leaving we met again with the first doctor we had seen the day before. In a grave voice, he informed us that Barry's cancer had at least a 50/50 chance of recurring.

Saturday morning we left Rochester dazed and confused. Three highly competent doctors offered three drastically different opinions. We wondered if the trip was even worth the trouble. Nonetheless, we decided to follow the last doctor's advice. For one, he was the only specialist in Barry's cancer. For another, no evidence of any cancer in Barry's body was visible at the moment, so we were probably best off simply to "wait and see."

The strain of those days was eased somewhat by two delicious dinners at Michael's, a downtown Rochester restaurant specializing in Greek cuisine. Avgolemono soup was my comfort food, just like my mother's home cooking. Under stressful circumstances, familiar foods were most welcome, a sign of normality when the rest of my world seemed to have gone awry. Barry ate ravenously. We also tried to calm down by walking at a nearby regional shopping center.

As Barry put it,

> Although we had never been mall-walkers before, the cold weather propelled us indoors. And simply escaping the medical environment was invigorating. Even I, who am by no means an aficionado of malls, enjoyed the diversion, if only to focus my eyes on anything other than medicine and doctors.

Weeks later, armed with our meticulous files, we battled with our HMO to be reimbursed for our $1500 fee for the Mayo Clinic. Were it not for help from both our parents, we could not have come up with all that money on the spot.

When our letters failed to produce positive results, we chose to take the matter up in person with our HMO appeals committee. Donning our best clothes—which for Barry meant his usual rumpled academic look—we pleaded our case before an intimidating group of 15 anonymous local citizens perched around a shiny conference table. We made a rather persuasive case, or so we thought.

But we persuaded nobody, and reimbursement was denied. It felt like failing my oral exams in graduate school, and it seemed as if the entire ordeal was a waste of time. Had we persisted, we could have taken our case up with the State of Illinois Consumer Services Board. But by then we had run out of steam. Fortunately the next year we had the opportunity to switch to a Preferred Provider Organization (PPO), and we did so. Barry changed his health plan out of necessity; I changed mine out of protest. We had both witnessed first-hand how our HMO treated us when we needed it most.

———•+•———

The day before Thanksgiving we had an appointment with another oncologist, Dr. Schmale, at Covenant Hospital in Champaign. A friend, whose late husband had had cancer, had recommended him.

"I've reviewed all your medical reports, and I'm sorry to tell you that because of the vascular invasion and the fact that your cancer was high-grade, there is a very strong possibility that it will recur," Dr. Schmale informed us.

"Just how sure are you?" Barry asked.

"About 90%," said Dr. Schmale.

"What do you suggest I do?"

"Let it go. You can't let this overwhelm your life. Just let it go."

How would Barry react to this latest dose of bad news?

> Needless to say, I was not reassured. On the other hand, I felt less confused than when I left Rochester a few weeks ago. At least now I had a better idea of what to expect. I braced myself for whatever my future would bring.
>
> My own stomach was once again turning in knots. It was not the best way to begin the Thanksgiving holiday.

The next day we enjoyed a bountiful holiday feast at the home of our friends, Sharon and Reed. It was the beginning of a tradition that would last several years. The tempting aromas of turkey permeated the entire house.

As Barry later reminisced,

> Celebrating this most American of all holidays with such a warm family was comforting. Although the past few months had been hell, that day felt like heaven.

We stayed home for the Christmas holidays, foregoing our usual trip to the Southwest to visit relatives. We needed some time to relax and unwind from the fall frenzy, and neither of us had the energy for a long trip. Barry's mother visited and a friend had invited the three of us for a potluck Christmas dinner party at her house. In light of all that had happened to us recently, this Christmas felt different from all others.

After all we had been through that fall, I couldn't help but wonder, "How many Christmases would Barry and I have left together?" That thought haunted me throughout the holiday season.

As we rang in the new year, we were both relieved to see 1993 come to an end. But would 1994 be any better? Who could tell?

———— • ————

During the months that followed, Barry continued to be monitored through a series of blood tests, CT-scans, and meetings with Dr. Johnson at Carle Clinic. The Carle Cancer Center is located in the basement. Even though we'd take a modern glass elevator to get there, I always felt as if we were sinking into the pits.

"Bad psychology. And terrible design," I said to myself every time I rode down that elevator.

To make matters worse, all the cancer patient examination rooms are in the basement, and none have windows. No visit to the Carle Cancer Center ever put me in a good mood, but the claustrophobic patient rooms made me feel even worse. Years later the Cancer Center was remodeled. Although the decor improved significantly, the exam rooms, chemotherapy lab, and radiation treatment center remain windowless.

On July 1, 1994 we both switched to our new health plan. We were no longer trapped in our HMO. Now if Barry needed to be treated elsewhere, we were finally free to go. The prison walls vanished.

Later that year, we enlisted the services of Patient Account Services (PAS), a Champaign company that helps consumers with health insurance claims. Richard Perry and his case manager, Rosalie Fuentes, run the office. A few friends had recommended PAS to us. At first I didn't see the need for such a service, but soon I would be proven wrong. Within weeks of switching to the PPO, what seemed like a mountain of medical bills, sometimes up to 40 pages per week, arrived at our doorstep. Despite its many faults, our HMO had shielded us from this mound of paperwork.

My attempts to question various medical charges were frustrating. At best, I would be transferred several times, reach a staff member's voice mail, leave our number, and wait for a call to be returned. At worst, I was cut off and forced to try all over again. Neither Barry nor I had the energy to deal with this constant series of run-arounds. We were feeling wiped out enough already.

Once we entered into an agreement with PAS, all this wasted effort was behind us. We simply copied off Barry's medical bills and sent them away. After reviewing our files and calling the health care providers on our behalf, PAS would inform us what the insurance had agreed to pay and what we really owed. Often we saw huge discrepancies between our initial bills and the final assessment that PAS had negotiated. Every few months PAS would send us spreadsheets providing an overview of all that had been paid and by whom. Over the years the firm saved us thousands of dollars and thousands of hours, and we were able to conserve our energy for more pressing tasks.

That summer the two of us made our pilgrimage to the West Coast to visit family and friends. It was Barry's "victory tour," the first time any of our California friends had seen us since he became ill. All were astonished at how well he looked and how much energy he had. In San Francisco, we hosted our annual picnic at the Palace of Fine Arts, a tradition we had started back in the early 1980's.

We rounded up our extended family of friends in the Bay Area. We had known most from graduate school at Berkeley's International House, but some went back even farther to my undergraduate days at Berkeley's Ida Sproul Hall. The Palace of Fine Arts is a relic from the

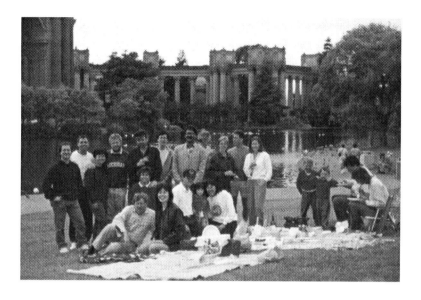

In the early 1980's we began our Fourth of July picnics at the Palace of Fine Arts with our extended family of Bay Area friends, a tradition that continued for over a decade. San Francisco, California; August 1995. (credit: Monica Chan)

1915 Panama Pacific Exposition, and its dramatic dome made a perfect backdrop for our annual photos. Usually the weather was cool, and sometimes the morning fog never even burned off. Nonetheless, no matter what the temperature, it was always one of our favorite days of the year. And this year the turnout was especially good.

As we drove south from Northern California we stopped overnight in San Luis Obispo at the infamous Madonna Inn, one of the quirkiest motels in the country. Each room has a unique décor, such as a honeymoon suite with pink velvet hearts, and a caveman theme with boulders surrounding the bathroom shower stall. We each peeked in the restaurant's men's room, a local tourist attraction which I had seen many times before, complete with rocks and waterfalls over the urinals. Staying there put us in the vacation spirit.

In Southern California we arrived in time for my cousin Jim's wedding, a great opportunity to reconnect with my many relatives from the Los Angeles area. I was especially pleased to see Jim's parents, Aunt Helen and Uncle Joe, with whom I had lived several years before. In many ways, they were almost like a second set of parents to me. Two of my aunts were visiting from the East Coast, and they joined us at the wedding. And it was the first time since Barry had been diagnosed that we saw my parents, my sister, Mary Anne, my brother-in-law, John, and their children. Jim and Debbie's wedding took place at St. Sophia's Greek Orthodox Cathedral in Los Angeles, and the reception was held at a grand old hotel in Hollywood. Both the bride and groom are musicians, and they had selected some terrific big band jazz music. Barry and I danced the night away. No matter what the rhythm, he danced to a beat of his own, most often at high-speed. Whether it was swing, disco, or free style, he usually wore me out. But given all he had been through, the fact that he could barely keep his feet on the ground was a good sign.

After the wedding, we spent several days with my family in Irvine and in La Jolla. Although it had only been about a year since I had seen them, it felt as if it had been much longer. It was good to get back home again.

That August I started my new job as Chair of the Building Research Council at our School of Architecture. I was looking forward to assuming a new role in the School. I felt fortunate as it was the first time this administrative role had been assigned to a woman. Half my position was teaching, which was by now old hat, but the administrative half was new. I quickly settled in to my research office at the south edge of campus, while keeping my old teaching office in the Architecture Building. I had always loved the latter, perched high atop the classic red brick, Georgian-style building. My huge south-facing dormer window brought a steady stream of sunshine into the room, making it feel almost like a greenhouse.

On September 13, 1994, Barry and I marked the one-year anniversary of the onset of his illness. So far nothing disastrous had happened.

"Could it be that this was really all just a bad dream, and that the cancer is all behind us?" I often wondered. "Maybe at last our lives are back to normal!"

But that was simply wishful thinking.

For just weeks later, in early October, a routine CT-scan revealed several spots on Barry's liver. Once again Felicia was visiting, and the two of us joined Barry for his appointment with Dr. Johnson. Dr.

Johnson displayed the large black and white negatives on the glass viewer.

"This time I see some spots on the liver," she said.

I darted out of my chair, and Barry and Felicia soon followed. We all studied the scans.

"Could these possibly be signs of fat in the liver?" Barry asked. "My brother has had that before, so maybe it runs in the family."

"Yes, but that's not very likely," the doctor replied.

She then scheduled Barry for an MRI and a needle aspiration biopsy. We would not know the results of all these tests for another few weeks.

On the afternoon of October 15, Dr. Johnson called Barry in his office, just minutes before he was about to teach his class.

"The lab tests results are in. The lesions in the liver are definitely cancerous," said Dr. Johnson.

How did Barry react?

> I was stunned. Even though my head was spinning, I managed to walk down the hall and into my classroom. I got through my class alright. But during my hour-long commute home I couldn't stop thinking about what this all meant—and how much time I had left.

It wasn't until after I arrived home from work that I learned the news from Felicia. While walking slowly down our steps, she told me that Barry had called home a while ago, after failing to reach me at work. Her voice was faint and she was on the verge of tears. In fact, we were all devastated.

Surely this was a turning point. The illness had now metastasized, and Barry technically had "advanced cancer." Who knows how much faster it could spin out of control?

We pulled ourselves together that evening in time to host two of our friends, Kaizad and Farzana. We had invited them over for dinner several days ago so that they could both enjoy our new deck.

As Barry later reflected,

> Kaizad was the man responsible for beautifying our
> landscape. Now he, along with his wife, brightened our spirits
> as well. Although both Kathy and I were preoccupied with the
> sudden turn of events, we managed to spend a normal evening
> together. Having company turned out to be just what the
> doctor ordered.

This most recent news was yet another blow, barely a year after the initial onslaught of the illness. The next week it all began to hit me. One sunny afternoon I sprawled out on a beach towel on our new deck. Within minutes tiny tear droplets began streaming down my cheeks. Soon I began to sob and just couldn't stop.

Somehow the words, "I want my Mommy," kept spinning over and over again in my head. At times I even said this Mantra out loud. I wanted my mother to help rescue me. Take care of me. Make it all better. But then reality set in: Mom was almost two thousand miles away. And even if she were here, there was little that she could do. It seemed that this time our situation might be hopeless. A few minutes later I ventured inside, lest any well-meaning passersby saw me in my sorry state. After a few days I managed to pull myself out of my melancholy mood.

"Kathy, snap out of it! Sinking deeper and deeper into depression can be debilitating. Stop wallowing in self-pity!" I kept telling myself. "And now, more than ever, you need to get re-energized. Don't waste any time. You need to move fast!"

I made my way back upstairs to Barry's cancer file, which had now grown to cover a large file cabinet. Retrieving all the information I had gathered last year, we began a barrage of phone calls and faxes to doctors across the country. The two of us called one of the doctors we had met at the Mayo Clinic, the doctor at Long Beach Medical Center from last year's CNN's "News from Medicine," as well as physicians at UCLA and the National Cancer Institute in Washington, DC.

When Barry informed the Mayo clinic physician about his latest news, the doctor said, "Well, this is serious."

"So what do you think I should do?" Barry asked.

"I don't know if I would do anything right now. You may just have to wait until it spreads to your lungs. Then it would be even more serious," the doctor said.

He implied that we were now at the stage where nothing much could be done. Needless to say, this was not encouraging. That was our final contact with Mayo Clinic.

The doctor from Long Beach stressed the value of chemosensitivity tests. Although we never did meet him in person, he reviewed Barry's medical records and was extremely helpful over the phone. He suggested that pieces of Barry's tumors be subjected to chemosensitivity tests in a lab to determine which treatments might be most effective.

"And get yourselves to the most aggressive liver surgeon you can find," he advised.

The next week we met with Dr. Johnson to discuss the implications of all this. In answer to our questions, she told us that most people who develop cancer in their liver have only months, not years, to live. In the meantime, she had checked with Dr. Tangen, the surgeon who operated on Barry last September. He was reluctant to perform surgery on Barry's liver largely because one of his tumors was quite close to the heart. Dr. Johnson added that chemotherapy was usually not effective in leiomyosarcoma patients. And she reminded us that the liver could only take a minimal amount of radiation, which would likely be ineffective. She confessed to us that at this juncture, she was not sure exactly what to do. Although we found it frustrating at the time, in retrospect, we both appreciated her candor. It was far better than having her feign expertise that she did not have. But by this time, we were convinced that we must now take matters into our own hands. For if we did not pursue other medical options, Barry, the historian, soon would be history.

Now that Mayo Clinic was out of the picture, I raised the possibility of traveling to MD Anderson Cancer Center in Houston, Texas. I mentioned Dr. Raphael Pollock, whose article on leiomyosarcoma I had read last autumn, and who was affiliated with that cancer center. As it turned out, Dr. Johnson and Dr. Pollock had been classmates in graduate school. She agreed that MD Anderson would be an excellent prospect.

Now another chapter in our medical odyssey was about to begin.

CHAPTER TWO

Lone Star Journeys
(1994 - 1995)

"...THE GREATER PART OF OUR HAPPINESS OR MISERY DEPENDS ON
OUR DISPOSITIONS AND NOT OUR CIRCUMSTANCES."
—MARTHA WASHINGTON

When Barry's cancer metastasized to his liver in October 1994, we knew that time would soon be running out. If, as Dr. Johnson had warned us, most patients in Barry's condition live only for months, we had no time to waste. My contacts from the previous year paid off. Dr. Raphael Pollock at the MD Anderson Cancer Center referred me to his colleague, Dr. Steven Curley. Dr. Curley was a specialist in treating leiomyosarcoma and as well as cancers in the liver. Over the phone, Dr. Curley sounded very pleasant, extremely competent, and relatively optimistic. He believed that even though Barry's cancer had metastasized, something could still be done, most likely through additional surgery. In contrast to our medical staff at Carle in Urbana, Dr. Curley examined many patients with leiomyosarcoma every year.

I was excited by my conversation with this new doctor. As soon as I hung up the phone, I called Barry at work. I felt relieved that I had found someone so knowledgeable and willing to help us—at last!

Shortly thereafter, I faxed Barry's medical documents to Dr. Curley, and he and Barry spoke by phone. The doctor then suggested that we travel to Houston to meet.

In November we embarked on what would be the first of five medical journeys to Texas. Since finances were tight, we decided to drive, with Barry's latest CT-scans and all his medical records carefully stowed in the back seat. We drove for three long days. Our first night on the road at Little Rock, Arkansas was marked by a disturbing incident.

During the pre-dawn hours while lying in bed at the Quality Inn, I was awakened from a deep sleep. A man was pounding on several doors, including our own.

"Come out! Come out! I know you're in there!" he screamed several times.

Suddenly I heard shattering glass, then horrific shrieks, then two men thrashing about the room beneath us. My heart was racing and my fingers were shaking as I dialed 911. Soon the police were on their way. In the meantime, it dawned on me that our precious medical documents were still lying on the back seat of our car.

"Could it be a rampage? Were thieves breaking into all the cars? How stupid we were to leave all Barry's records in the car! Now they'll all be stolen!" I said to myself.

Within minutes sirens began blowing and red lights started flashing outside our window. It sounded as if the police were hauling someone away. When the commotion was over, I was relieved to find our car unscathed. But my adrenaline level was so high that I could not fall back asleep. Later I learned from the motel receptionist that this had been a classic three-way lover's quarrel. Although I had been preoccupied with our own medical troubles, the next day all I could think about was that violent scene.

"Forget about the cancer! We both could have been killed!" I said to Barry several times that day.

By now I felt lucky just to be alive.

That day we visited President Clinton's hometown of Hope, Arkansas, stopping to take some photos in front of Clinton's boyhood home and to visit the local museum. We even ran into one of the President's cousins, an elderly woman sporting a Bill Clinton T-shirt.

We struck up a conversation with the women working in the gift shop

"So where are you two from, and what are you doing down here? Are you on vacation?" one of them asked.

"We're driving down to Texas for a visit," I replied.

It was far easier than explaining our medical saga. How I wished that we really had been on a vacation!

When we arrived in Houston on the afternoon of November 3, we headed straight for the Jesse H. Jones Rotary House International. This facility, right across the street from MD Anderson Cancer Center, was built in the early 1990's for cancer patients and their families.

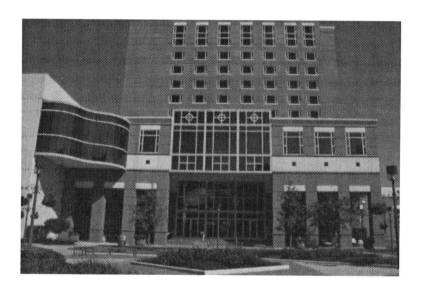

For a year the Jesse H. Jones Rotary House International at the University of Texas MD Anderson Cancer Center became our home away from home. We stayed there five times, including two weeks during the holiday season. Houston, Texas; October 1994. (credit: author)

The accommodations were stunning. Rotary House caters to patients' and families' every need: from its bright atrium, to its sun-drenched indoor swimming pool and exercise room, to its attractive restaurant and deli. It also features a lounge, library and information center with an extensive collection of books, pamphlets, and videos. Part of it is set aside as a "Laughter Library." Here residents can check out comedy films and watch them in their rooms, each complete with its own video cassette player. A bag full of popcorn awaited us in our room. The pastel pink and peach decor, complete with a small kitchenette, dishes, silverware, a microwave oven, small refrigerator, and even a dishwasher, were most welcome. Soon after our arrival, staff members oriented us around the facility. We were in awe of our gorgeous surroundings—a far cry from the Quality Inn of a few nights before.

The next day, prior to meeting with Dr. Steven Curley, we were introduced to our Patient Care Coordinator, our social worker, and our Patient Accounts Representative. They were all extremely solicitous and answered all our questions. MD Anderson was making a terrific first impression.

Later that morning we had a productive hour-long session with Dr. Curley and his assistant. The doctor struck us as extremely knowledgeable, patient, and thoroughly in command of the situation. At the same time he fielded every question that we asked, and we had plenty. He described how the surgery on Barry's liver would proceed. He planned on meeting us one more time later that afternoon, but was unable to due to an emergency. Instead, the next day he met us for an early breakfast at the Rotary House, just before we left town. At that time, he pulled out his appointment book and scheduled the upcoming operation for December 8, 1994. Our trip would coincide with the holiday season, not the best time to endure a stressful, high-risk cancer operation.

During our stay at Rotary House, we also met Steve Thorney, a minister, and Sister Alice Potts. Sister Alice ran a weekly support group for cancer patients and their families, along with a Well Wives Club. We attended one of these support groups where a young woman tearfully recounted how her husband had been savaged by a fierce brain tumor. It was probably to be the last Christmas her family would have all together. Upon hearing her tale, most of the group members were in tears. I, too, was moved by her plight, realizing that many others had cases far worse than ours. However, Barry found the session more depressing than helpful. It was one of the few support groups we attended.

While in Houston, I took advantage of the expertise across the street and made an appointment for a head-to-toe cancer check for myself. It struck me as a good opportunity for some preventive medicine. The nurse who examined me said that all looked good. She suggested I get a mammogram once every year or two, and that I be checked annually by a dermatologist for skin cancer.

We returned to Urbana for just another few weeks. During this time, Barry reached another milestone: his 40th birthday. Just a year ago, I wondered if he would even reach the big 4-0. Now that he had made it, it was a reason to celebrate. I had wanted to throw a surprise party for him, as many of our friends had done for their spouses, but after our trip to Texas, my energy was sapped. So when our friend Norma volunteered to host the festivities at her house, I jumped at the chance. She even repeated the offer a year later, and we took her up on it then as well. Some close friends joined us, and we all split our favorite Chicago-style pizza. Although the mood was jovial, I couldn't help but ponder the inevitable: would Barry's 40th birthday be his last?

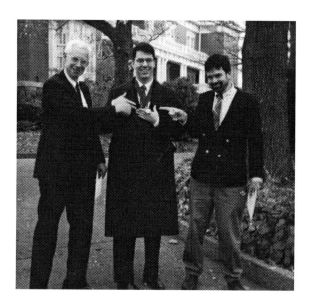

Colleague Herbert Lasky, Eastern Illinois University honor student Jeff Waldhoff, and Barry at a special awards ceremony held at the Governor's Mansion. Springfield, Illinois; November 1994. (credit: author)

Soon it was time to drive back to Texas for Barry's operation. Barry delegated his teaching duties to several graduate students, and for the first time ever, he composed objective tests for his final exams. His colleagues were supportive as ever, and did not appear to begrudge his taking an early leave. I, too, ended my semester a week early in order to drive down to Houston.

Early one December Saturday morning, Barry and I squeezed in our last suitcase and slammed the trunk for the last time. Our car was jam-packed with an odd assortment of clothes, books, snacks, Christmas presents, and a 12-pack of Diet Coke. Simply preparing for the trip had left me exhausted. Just hours before we had finished grading piles of students' projects, paying a slew of bills, and taking care of what seemed like hundreds of last-minute items at home. We even dashed off all our holiday greeting cards to over 100 friends and family, notifying them of Barry's upcoming surgery. We inched out of our driveway onto Pennsylvania Avenue. I was crying so hard that I could barely see as we drove down our street.

"What if this turned out to be a one-way trip for Barry?" I wondered. "Would I have to drive back alone?"

Nevertheless, I was heartened by the fact that at least the weather cooperated. As we drove straight south on I-55 through Illinois, Missouri, Arkansas, and Mississippi, and finally out of the Snowbelt, the danger of winter weather was soon behind us. We made a detour at Lambert's, Home of "Throwed Rolls," an establishment which advertised on huge billboards from over 50 miles away. My students had told us not to miss it. Customers wait outside in a long line, only to be greeted by servers throwing hot rolls across the dining room. Somehow we managed to catch most of the rolls tossed in our direction. It was a festive atmosphere, and for a few moments we almost forgot where we were going and why.

Our first night we stopped near Jackson, Mississippi, where we spotted a Pizza Hut off the freeway. All was fine until we asked the waitress for some oregano to spice up the meal.

"Regano? What's that? Pepper or something?" she asked with her southern twang.

Incredible as it seemed, she had never heard of oregano before. Barry compared it to a student not knowing what a teacher was. We laughed about this mishap several times as we continued our drive south.

Our next stop was in New Orleans, one of our favorite cities. Within minutes of checking into our historic hotel on the edge of the French Quarter, we enjoyed a gargantuan buffet lunch at the famed Court of Two Sisters. There, several years before, Barry and one of my colleagues, Jim, had squared off in an eating contest. Brunch lasted from about 11 a.m. to 2 p.m., and Barry and Jim had been feasting away at the buffet almost all that time—with seconds, thirds, and possibly even fourths. This time we made up for our high caloric intake by weaving our way through several miles of nooks and crannies in the French Quarter. That evening we drove out to City Park where we saw one of the most spectacular Christmas light displays ever. The next morning we enjoyed beignets at Cafe du Monde, where we purchased a tape, "Sidewinder Duo," from two sidewalk jazz musicians who entertained us. We played one of their songs, "I Can Make You Laugh", over and over again in our car for the remainder of the trip. In 24 hours we packed in about as much of New Orleans as possible. The revelry of this festive city took our minds off our troubles, if only for a day. My pessimism was put temporarily at bay.

Upon arriving in Houston, we checked in once again at the Rotary House. Having stayed there just a month earlier, it already looked familiar to us. It was a welcome sight. In many ways, it already had become our home away from home. We even found three Christmas cards awaiting us at Rotary House. Our efforts to alert friends and relatives about our whereabouts during the holidays had already paid off. Within days, a flood of cards began pouring in, buoying our spirits at an extraordinarily stressful time. Later that day, Barry's mother, Felicia, arrived from Phoenix.

The next morning the three of us met with several physicians about Barry's upcoming operation. The anesthesiologist tried to reassure us.

"Stop to think about it," he said. "Your drive down to Houston was actually more dangerous than Barry's upcoming operation! Before you know it, it will be over".

Soon afterwards, we met with Dr. Curley.

As Barry recalled,

> By now I was salivating over the prospect of eating at my
> favorite local Thai restaurant in nearby Rice Village. However,
> Dr. Curley adeptly played the part of the killjoy, informing me
> that in preparation for the next day's surgery, I could not eat
> for the rest of the day. To make matters worse, he ordered me
> to drink 15 glasses of what looked like arsenic. Kathy walked
> over to the MD Anderson pharmacy to pick up the drink, and
> lugged the heavy containers across the overpass to Rotary
> House. The purpose of all those drinks was to empty my
> gastrointestinal tract. The strategy worked, but it was not a
> procedure that I would recommend to others. My wife and my
> mother left me alone in our hotel room for part of the evening
> while I raced back and forth to the bathroom.
>
> When they returned to our room, the three of us watched
> a video to put us all at ease. The film was *The Desperate Hours,*
> about three escaped convicts who terrorize a suburban
> midwestern family in the 1950's, and it starred Frederic March
> and Humphrey Bogart. It was one of Bogart's last films.
> Despite the tense plot, it actually relaxed me, and I had a good
> night's sleep. In contrast to my first operation, I was completely
> calm before my surgery at MD Anderson.

Before dawn the next day the three of us walked together across the
skyway to the hospital. While the passageway had been full of foot
traffic by day, at this time of the morning we were alone. It was eerie.
Our first meeting was with a charming French anesthesiologist. Again
he reassured us about all that was to take place. We chatted briefly
about La Jolla and the University of California at San Diego, two places
we all knew well. We then escorted Barry to the locker room, where he
was again transformed from a person into a patient. Leaving his street
clothes behind, he donned the hospital attire. A surgical gown covered
his body, an odd-looking cap enveloped his jet-black hair, and Ted hose
were wrapped tightly around his legs to keep his circulation moving. It
was definitely not the Barry I knew. As the transporters whisked him
away, we gave him a good-bye kiss and wished him good luck.

On the one hand, this episode was less traumatic than Barry's first operation. Instead of an emergency, it was all planned in advance. Yet on the other hand, this time we had traveled hundreds of miles, invested thousands of dollars, and spent so much energy preparing for this journey that the sight of Barry being wheeled away on his gurney almost made me cave in to my emotions. Nonetheless I tried my best to hide behind a cheerful facade.

Felicia and I staked out a comfortable spot in the surgical waiting area. Dr. Curley had informed us that Barry's operation would take anywhere from four to eight hours. So we were prepared for a long day. Now a veteran of prolonged hospital stays, this time I came prepared with plenty of books and music. I had hoped that my songs from the Greek islands and my favorite holiday music would cheer me up. The waiting room was crowded. Soon after we settled in, almost every spot was taken. As I scanned the room I noticed that the eyes of many of those around me were red and swollen. Some people could barely stay awake. And some, perched atop their suitcases, must have just arrived from the airport.

Several tall snake plants surrounded the waiting area, setting it off from the adjacent corridor. When I asked about them, one of the nurses told me that the plants had been placed there intentionally in order to give the patients' families a greater sense of privacy.

"What a great idea!" I thought. "At a time like this, some of us need to hide."

I also noticed the conspicuous absence of a television. The nurse later informed me that this, too, was deliberate. Apparently the surgical area used to have them, but the staff observed that the music, plots, and mood of certain TV shows triggered the visitors' emotions. So they removed all TVs.

"We came to the conclusion that in a setting like this, television can do more harm than good," she informed me.

"Right on," I agreed.

After a couple hours, the receptionist announced, "Mrs. Riccio. You have a phone call!"

The disruption startled me, and I wondered who would track me down here of all places. It turned out to be our good friend, Barbara from Oregon. She had introduced Barry and me back in 1976 while we were all graduate students at Berkeley's International House. I hadn't spoken with her in months. Her voice was breaking.

"You two have been through so much together," she said. "I can't believe it. And now this!"

We chatted for about five minutes, when the receptionist summoned me once again.

"Dr. Curley's nurse wants to speak with you," she whispered.

"I have to go, Barbara. I'll try to get back to you later," I said as I rushed to hang up the phone.

By now my heart was beating so quickly that I could almost hear it. I glanced at the clock. Only two and one half-hours had passed.

"It's too soon for Barry's operation to be over," I said to myself. "Something must have gone wrong!"

"The operation has ended," said the nurse. "Dr. Curley will be out shortly to speak with you."

Even though her voice sounded calm, I could feel my own legs shaking. I could barely stand up. In a few minutes, Dr. Curley and a nurse arrived. They asked us to meet them in a separate consultation room, that famous signal that something had gone awry.

"The operation was only partially successful," he informed us. "I was able to remove only a small portion of the cancer eating away at Barry's liver. I cut out about half of Barry's tumors and only about 1% of Barry's liver, but only one-quarter of the cancer mass in the liver. The rest of the cancer is still there."

No sooner had Dr. Curley spoken than Felicia burst into tears. The nurse put her arm around her in an effort to console her. And while I could feel my heart skip a few beats, I tried my best to maintain my composure by asking questions and taking notes. My Uncle Peter's advice echoed in my mind.

"Will you tell Barry, or should we?" I asked.

"I'll tell him," Dr. Curley said, "That's my job."

After meeting with the doctor, I dragged myself down the hall to phone my parents, who had been awaiting the news in San Diego. I asked them to call a few others. At that point I didn't feel up to talking with anyone else. Felicia and I waited for several more hours until Barry left the recovery room and checked into his hospital room. This time it was a private room, and I was relieved to see that Barry had no roommate. I later learned that most rooms at MD Anderson's hospital were private due to the severity of the patients' conditions. By the time we saw Barry later that afternoon it was almost dark. He was lying in his hospital bed, with an eerie fluorescent light shining on his face. He looked exceptionally pale and his eyes seemed to have lost their sparkle. Perhaps he was simply exhausted from the surgery.

"He looks just like Jesus Christ!" his mother gasped.

"Do you know what happened during the operation?" I asked Barry.

I was hoping that the doctor had already broken the bad news.

"Dr. Curley told me that he couldn't remove most of the cancer," he explained, "But he said that in some ways that's o.k., because now it will be easier to track the tumors with chemotherapy."

Much to my surprise, Barry seemed unaffected by the news. As he later recalled,

> Perhaps the doctor was simply putting a positive spin on things, but nonetheless, I found his comments reassuring. In fact, I was only slightly disappointed.

We stayed with Barry in his room for a few hours, and then left him to catch up on his sleep.

Later that evening when we arrived back at our room at the Rotary House, both Felicia and I were devastated by all the day's events. She would not stop sobbing, and watching her in that state made me feel even worse.

I felt like a stampede of elephants had stomped all over me. Every bone in my body was aching, and my head was reeling. Yet I tried to keep from breaking down. I had cried so much in the past, and I knew that once I started I couldn't stop. While some people find crying to be cathartic, it made me feel worse. My contact lenses would become so blurry that I couldn't even see, and my nose so stuffed that I could hardly breathe. I soon began to wonder whether or not it was a good idea to be sharing the hotel room with Felicia alone for the next several days. Unfortunately, Barry and I could not afford to rent a room all to ourselves for two weeks.

The day after Barry's operation I sent out a fax to our colleagues notifying them about the partly failed operation. The response to our communication was phenomenal. Just about every day for the next few weeks, we received cards, letters, faxes, phone calls, and flowers from family and friends across the country. And the Christmas cards continued to pour in. Several called Barry directly in his hospital room. He had lengthy discussions with each of them. For instance, with our friend, Kate Harrison, Barry was engrossed in a political conversation about Newt Gingrich and the recent Republican party triumph in Congress. At times the staff at the nursing station had to take messages for him while he was on the phone with someone else. While one would think that all this activity would have worn Barry out, instead it energized him.

One of the highlights of my day was opening up our mail at the Rotary House and bringing it over to the hospital to show Barry. Hearing from the outside world was a reminder that life was simply going on. For example, two friends of ours, Karen and Alex, even sent us a fax announcing the birth of their new baby. Several gifts surprised us, too. One of my favorites was a tiny Christmas tree full of handmade seashell ornaments. My friends Betsey and Craig had sent it to us all the way from Cincinnati. As high school students in La Jolla, Betsey and I had spent many pleasant days together with friends near the beach. Opening up the Christmas tree triggered a slew of happy memories. Another of my favorite gifts was a heaping basket of fruit sent by my four cousins in New England, George, Norah, Jon, and Mary. Although Barry couldn't eat them at the time, they provided a healthy snack for Felicia and me while in the hospital room. Yet another surprise gift that arrived at the Rotary House was a stuffed animal, a duckbill platypus. Our friends, Walter and Charlotte, sent it from Urbana, and it came in handy. For weeks Barry clutched the platypus whenever he sneezed or laughed, two motions that were quite painful after his abdominal surgery. Knowing that so many people were rooting for us was heartening. It was the perfect antidote to the backdrop of Christmas carols and holiday décor that accompanied us throughout the cancer center—well meaning but vain attempts to cheer up people like me.

Almost every night Felicia and I sat in the Rotary House lobby for several hours listening to holiday entertainment. The atrium was decorated to the hilt for Christmas, with a huge tree overflowing with colorful ornaments. Here as well as in the clinic, costumed carolers sang out the familiar holiday tunes. I was extremely grateful for the distraction and the chance to escape from our hotel room. Yet I was in a fragile emotional state. I soon discovered that I was over-reacting to what I heard. Songs with a quick beat like "Let it Snow" and "Sleigh Ride" were uplifting, but more somber pieces like "Silent Night" and "Oh Little Town of Bethlehem" unleashed a flood of tears.

"What on earth are we doing here at this time of year?" I constantly asked myself. "Everyone at home is celebrating at holiday parties. But here we are stuck in Houston, far away from our friends and family!"

Every once in a while when I started feeling sorry for myself, I kept trying to snap out of it. Sometimes I did, but sometimes I didn't. I was especially touched by a group of local school children who sang international holiday music. I even recognized "Silent Night" in Greek. My favorite group played Latin American jazz. Their songs were not even reminiscent of the holiday season, but spirited enough to take me to another place and time.

Felicia and I spent one evening at the Rotary House with a Well Wives support group facilitated by Sister Alice. The session was gut-wrenching. One of the women described in graphic detail her husband's operation that had taken place that same day. In her case, as well as in ours, doctors had to cut the surgery short. They found that tiny grains of cancer had already spread throughout her husband's body, sewed him back up, and sent him home. Now they were at the end of their rope, and nothing more could be done. Others in the group told equally depressing tales. When placed in perspective, our own situation didn't look quite so bleak.

In addition to the support group, another outlet for me was exercise. I have long been an avid swimmer, and the glistening pool at the Rotary House beckoned me every morning. As soon as I got out of bed, I put on my bathing suit and went down the elevator for a swim. I swam half a mile in half an hour, and if I had time, I made a brief detour to the Jacuzzi. While I was in the water, I felt like a different person. There, while immersed in the rhythm of my strokes and kicks, I couldn't cry. And for a few moments I almost forgot where I was. The pool became my salvation.

The weekend after Barry's operation, Peter, one of his best friends from graduate school days arrived from the Bay Area. I was so relieved to see a familiar face in this unfamiliar place. I met Peter in the lobby of Rotary House that morning and escorted him across the skyway to find Barry in the hospital. Watching these two meet under such unusual circumstances moved me, and I realized how powerful a force friendship can be. Barry was buoyed by his visit. Peter spent hours at Barry's bedside, discussing his medical situation, academia, and politics. He joined us for a meeting with Dr. Curley. He asked questions about Barry's illness and was impressed with the doctor's expertise. When the weekend was over, Peter returned to Stanford to grade his final exams. It was a tribute to Barry that he had flown so far just to see him, in the midst of such a busy schedule.

The next week when Barry was released from the hospital, my cousin, Jack, flew in from Maine.

"I'm so glad you're here!" I said when I greeted him. "You're giving us the best possible Christmas present!"

Prior to Jack's arrival, the only time I felt up to driving was during one brief outing for lunch with Peter and Felicia in nearby Rice Village. For days our car had sat untouched in the parking lot. Well after Barry's surgery, I still felt jittery. Like a little old lady, I feared getting in an accident if I drove anywhere at all.

Jack arrived just in time. An accomplished traveler and a preservation buff, he rented a car and drove us all around Houston. Venturing out of the MD Anderson complex felt good. Even though we all loved our accommodations at Rotary House where the staff catered to our every need, we relished the chance to escape to a normal place. We concentrated on the historical part of the city. Here a stunning group of Victorian homes, all decked out for Christmas, was dwarfed by monstrous skyscrapers only a few blocks away. Rarely had we seen such a jarring juxtaposition of old and new architecture, but it was a sight worth seeing.

When we returned from our excursion, we found a surprise: my other cousin, Andoni, had flown in for a short visit from Dallas.

Soon afterwards, Jack returned home to snowy Maine, and we, too, prepared to leave Houston. I was sad to say good-bye to Jack but eternally grateful for his visit. We had our final meeting with Dr. Curley and agreed that we would contact him again from Arizona around the new year. At that time he would have completed various chemosensitivity tests to see what combination of chemicals, if any, appeared to be most aggressive in shrinking Barry's liver tumors.

A few days later, we began our journey to Arizona to celebrate the holidays with the Riccios. Once again we struggled to stuff all our worldly goods back into our Honda. Plus now we had an additional passenger: Felicia, and her luggage. But somehow we managed. I felt pangs of pain as we left the Rotary House. After two weeks, the place had begun to feel like home. In an odd way, our car, too, evoked the same sensation. Its cheerful jade exterior, its soft tan seats, and even our Illinois license plates were comforting to me.

"Maybe that's what gypsies and vagabonds feel like," I wondered. "Without a real house, your few worldly goods become your temporary home. A strange feeling...."

I pondered these thoughts as we drove off around noontime, heading west.

As we made our way out of the Houston metroplex, we reconnected with the never-ending Interstate 10 and its 880 miles across the state of Texas. For me, it was going to be an exceptionally long ride since Barry was under doctor's orders not to drive. I pressed the pedal to the metal.

"The faster you drive, the sooner you'll get there," I told myself.

Our first stop was San Antonio, only three hours away. We checked into the Marriott at River Center, a hotel Barry and I had admired during two recent visits, but at which we had never stayed. Our room overlooked the historic Riverwalk. That evening we got together with Carole, an old friend of ours from Berkeley's International House. It was wonderful to see her smiling face waiting for us in the lobby of our hotel.

"You've been through a lot since I last saw you," she said as she greeted us.

"To hell and back, it seems," I said. "But it's great to be back in the real world once again."

After dinner with Carole, Felicia went upstairs to rest while the three of us went for a boat ride together along the San Antonio River. Just a few days before, Felicia had asked Dr. Curley if Barry could handle the boat ride, but the doctor reassured us that this was no problem. In fact, the river is so narrow and so calm that one barely senses being on the water; it's about as far from a boating experience on the rough seas as one can get. With thousands of holiday lights draped over trees and bridges, and their reflections glistening in the water, the city sparkled. Never had we seen San Antonio look like this. It was just what the doctor ordered, a welcome change from the medical scene in which we had been held captive for so long.

The next morning we drove back onto Interstate 10 and began our marathon ride across the great state of Texas. This leg of the trip was just about as long as our journey from Illinois to Texas, only every mile we drove further west was even further from home. We were all pleasantly surprised to find the Lone Star State much more scenic than we had expected. Through much of our ride, we could see panoramic rolling hills and jagged mountains sat off in the distance, complementing our "Under the Western Sky" cowboy music that we played in our car. My favorite Frank Sinatra songs also entertained us. "I Get a Kick out of You," "Fly Me to the Moon," and "I've Got You Under My Skin," kept me wide-awake.

As we wove our way through El Paso we were surprised to see Mexico just across the freeway.

"Now we have really come far from home," I thought. "We can't get much farther south than this."

We stopped overnight in Las Cruces, New Mexico. The next day as we began our final leg through the desert, we made a brief detour in Tucson, Arizona, to visit some friends. On December 23, we arrived in the Phoenix area just after sunset and in time for the evening rush hour. After so much driving, I was utterly exhausted.

Two days later we celebrated Christmas at the home of Greg and Maria, Barry's brother and sister-in-law. Maria made her famous antipasto with green beans, olives, tomatoes, onions, and peppers. Whenever we were in Arizona for the holidays, she always gave us a jar of it to take back to Illinois. It was fun to be around the family again, especially the kids who were running around the house playing with their brand new Christmas toys. Scottsdale seemed especially cheerful at this time of year. The warm, sunny days and crisp desert nights brought a special feel to the air.

One of the highlights of our Arizona stay was a visit from our friend, Mary Nicholas. She had worked with Barry in the Internal Revenue Service over a dozen years ago, and the three of us have been friends ever since. She drove from Orange County, California, all the way to Phoenix just to see us. The three of us took a day trip up to Sedona and points north, where we had lunch at a scenic restaurant overlooking the river in Oak Creek Canyon. We enjoyed seeing the San Francisco peaks all covered in snow. In late afternoon we went hiking at Red Rock State Park. I was concerned about Barry exerting himself just on the heels of his surgery, but he did surprisingly well. The rugged mountains formed a dramatic silhouette against the brilliant desert sunset. The stunning scenery made me realize how lucky we all were simply to be alive.

While in Arizona, Barry telephoned Dr. Curley about the results of the chemosensitivity tests performed on the cancerous tumors removed from his liver. Dr. Curley sounded more optimistic than we expected.

"I've identified a combination of drugs that looks potentially promising. Their side effects would be relatively mild," he said to Barry. "You can begin chemotherapy at the end of January under Dr. Johnson's supervision in Urbana."

Dr. Curley also informed Barry that his tumor was somewhat rational in its behavior, and that its doubling time was only moderate. His tumors would take at least six months to double in size. This gave us more time to work with. Although I dreaded the thought of Barry undergoing chemotherapy, he actually looked forward to it.

"At least something more can be done," he explained.

The day after New Year's we began our long drive back home to Illinois. By the first night we reached Albuquerque, and the second night we made it to Amarillo. The next morning, we made a cameo appearance at The Big Texan, a well-known eatery off I-40 that advertises on giant billboards for miles and miles in either direction, even as far away as Joplin, Missouri. We wanted to stop by for old time's sake, as for years Barry had regaled me with his misadventure there:

> My appetite was at one time legendary. In the summer of
> 1973, as my mother and I were making our way across the
> country in order to meet my father in Phoenix, we stopped off

at a place called The Big Texan in Amarillo, Texas. It was a somewhat hokey place, but I was seduced into playing their big game, namely devouring an entire 72 ounce steak, baked beans, a potato, and a soda, all within one hour—and without leaving the table. The draw was that if you could perform this feat, you would not have to pay a penny for the meal. But the catch was that if you couldn't, the meal would cost $13, a not insubstantial sum, especially to one who was only 18 years of age.

I made a valiant effort and in the first half-hour, I really thought I would win the battle. But as the clock ticked away, the challenge became more and more formidable. And 45 minutes into the hour, after chewing the same piece of meat for nearly 10 minutes, I wearily raised the white flag of surrender. Needless to say I had to pay for this debacle with my own money. But there was one consolation prize. And that was that we could take the meat with us on our trip. The next day we had it for lunch, and it tasted much, much better.

The contest is still being held. The restaurant touts its record-holders: one hearty eater who devoured his steak in less than nine minutes, and another who downed not just one, but two 72-ounce steaks in an hour. All the contest memorabilia as well as the gift shop fascinated me. There I purchased two clear plastic glasses shaped like cowboy boots. When we got home, I enjoyed pouring orange juice in them for breakfast, a touch of the Wild West to start the day. We also bought a videotape about the legendary Route 66, featuring The Big Texan. But after glancing out the gift shop window, we could see that snow was already beginning to fall. Wanting to avoid the snowstorm, we raced back into our car and continued east. Two days later we arrived in Illinois. And after our month-long journey, we were relieved to be home.

Soon afterwards we both resumed teaching. That spring semester Barry was full-time at EIU and part-time at U of I. This would be his last term at the U of I, as teaching nine classes a year was getting exhausting. His courses that school year included American Constitutional History, surveys in Pre- and Post-Civil War America, historical methods, and various graduate seminars on American Political Thought and Culture. In a typical semester he had between 120 and 140 students, and except for December 1994, when we left for Texas, he did virtually all the grading himself. This would include take-home essay exams, final exams, term papers, a series of smaller writing assignments, and extra credit book reviews. It seemed like he always had a huge stack of student papers to review. In his early years at EIU, his teaching schedule often spanned 12 hours per day. Sometimes he would leave our house at 9:30 in the morning and not return until almost midnight. Now that he was about to be on chemotherapy, something had to give.

Several people came to Barry's rescue that winter. One was a graduate assistant at EIU who showed films during the weeks that Barry had to take off for treatment. Another was our friend, Mark, a history professor at the U of I, who substituted for Barry's class there on at least eight occasions. In addition, many of Barry's EIU colleagues took over his lecture classes.

Entertainment also came to Barry's rescue. No sooner would he leave the chemotherapy lab than he would stop by Blockbuster Video to rent a film. Most of the movies he chose were from the 1950's, since these were the ones he had grown up on: *Picnic* (with William Holden), *Anatomy of a Murder* (Jimmy Stewart), *The Bad Seed* (Patty McCormick) and *Marty* (Ernest Borgnine). Once in a while he selected some more recent films, such as *Birdman of Alcatraz* (Burt Lancaster), and *Unforgiven* (a psychological Western directed and acted by Clint Eastwood).

In late January 1995, Barry began chemotherapy at Carle Hospital in Urbana. His treatments consisted of a mixture of 5-FU (5 fluorouracil) and interferon. That involved roughly 45 minutes to one-hour visits to the hospital five days a week for the first week for the 5-FU and interferon; and then five-minute visits to the hospital three days a week during the second week just for the interferon. The remaining two weeks of the month, Barry was not obliged to go to the hospital or clinic. He continued teaching three out of four weeks, including the week when he was given only the interferon. He continued this regimen from January until April, a total of 12 rounds. The cycle was then repeated from May until July.

The morning when he began his chemotherapy, I took off from work to be with Barry. I met with the nurses and watched as the drug was first administered. Oddly enough, that afternoon I started to ache all over. I must have talked myself into it after imagining what all these drugs were doing to Barry.

Here is what he recalled.

> At 3:30 that afternoon, I began to feel tired and flushed. Later in the day, I began to ache and took a nap. Ironically, I began feeling the side effects while reading about them in the vast notebook that the Carle nurses had given me. But after some time, I was convinced that the side effects I was feeling were not psychosomatic. They continued for the rest of the week. Nonetheless, I found them tolerable largely because of Tylenol. The next week, when I returned to teaching, I started to feel worse. I began to experience diarrhea, but soon it went away.
>
> One Saturday night in February, the day after my first two-week round of treatment was completed, I was unable to sleep. I was experiencing intense and yet diffuse back pain. For about 20 minutes, I was drenched in a cold sweat. Even Tylenol didn't help. The pain eventually subsided, but the next afternoon, while watching "The McLaughlin Group" on TV, the same thing happened. I began to worry, but, fortunately, the rest of the day I felt much better.

Just before Barry's second round of chemotherapy, our friend Peter flew out to visit us from California. After having seen him in Texas only a few months ago, Peter was astounded at Barry's vigorous appearance. Just before Peter returned for the West Coast, the three of us met with Dr. Johnson. Since Peter had joined us for an appointment with Dr. Curley in Houston, he wanted to meet Barry's local doctor in Urbana as well.

During that time Barry came down with a mild cold. Soon afterwards, Barry began noticing that his eyes were smaller than usual and severely bloodshot. The next morning he could hardly open them. A thick, heavy crust had formed over his eyelids. It took him 10 minutes to remove this overlay and open his eyes. To make matters worse, within a day, Barry's face began hurting immensely. His cheeks turned a deep purple.

"It felt as if someone placed a hot iron upon my cheeks," he said. "I look like an AIDS patient, far worse than Tom Hanks in the famous film *Philadelphia*."

We were both frightened. First, Barry went to see his general practitioner. He prescribed antibiotics which, unfortunately, did nothing. Later Barry saw an ophthalmologist. He diagnosed Barry as having conjunctivitis which worsened into blepharitis, and he pre-scribed some pills and gave Barry an ointment to apply to his cheeks. Almost immediately, Barry began to feel some relief. He had to stay home from school for another few days until the symptoms subsided.

In the middle of Barry's second round of treatment, around Valentine's Day, Barry's nose began to bleed. He initially suspected that it was because of the cold, dry air. We had spent a fair amount of time outside while visiting nearby Amish country with a friend. But it soon became clear that the bloody nose was yet another side effect of his chemotherapy. He soon experienced sores in his mouth and bleeding as well. One morning I woke up to a foul-smelling stench. It turned out to be dried blood that had caked onto Barry's lips. By now it seemed like everything that could possibly go wrong was going wrong. And this was the supposedly mild form of chemotherapy!

In April, Barry finally had an interview for a tenure-track position at EIU, the type of job he had been craving for a decade. The night before, Barry's hemorrhoids began to bother him immensely. He squirmed while struggling to sit on a living room chair. Later that night, Barry drove to Charleston to sleep at a motel near the university, as his interview was scheduled at 8 a.m., and he wanted to make sure he was there on time. The hemorrhoidal pain was so intense while he was driving down to Charleston that at times, he was forced to partially stand up while at the steering wheel. Barry tossed and turned in his motel bed, but finally, perhaps because of all the exertion, he sweated himself to sleep. The next morning the pain was much less severe. Because he was so exhausted, Barry was actually fairly relaxed during his job interview. And after having taught there on a temporary basis for several years, he already knew everyone in the department. The inter-view went smoothly. Shortly thereafter, Barry discovered that among the 65 or so applicants, he was the department's top choice. Within a month, Barry was offered the tenure-track job. Barry's longtime dream had now been fulfilled. His quest, since he had received his Ph.D. over 10 years ago, had finally come to an end.

———————

Three more trips to Texas followed that year. In contrast to our previous visits, we decided to fly down. Our May trip provided a temporary respite, as the CT-scan revealed that Barry's tumors had begun to shrink by nearly one-third. The chemotherapy seemed to be working. We were elated! My parents had flown out from California to Houston to join us, and we celebrated together. During their visit, I shot a dramatic photo of Barry running through the Cancer Survivors' Plaza. And between medical appointments one afternoon, we squeezed in a visit to the historic section of Galveston.

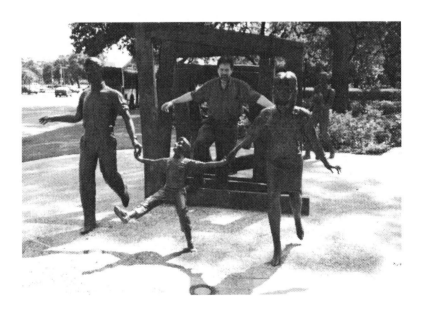

Barry at Cancer Survivor's Plaza. Houston, Texas; May 1995. (credit: author)

Both Mom and Dad were surprised to see how Barry's appearance had changed. Due to his chemotherapy, his thick head of hair had been reduced to a patchy veil barely covering his scalp. His beard had thinned out and his eyebrows had almost disappeared. To them, he looked like a different person. Since I had seen him every day, his

transformation seemed less dramatic to me. However, since the chemotherapy turned out to be successful, it was a small price to pay. And the
good news overshadowed all else.

I continued to swim every day at the Rotary House pool. Once
again it had become my home away from home, my escape. The sun
was streaming in, the turquoise waters were glistening, and in stark
contrast to the sultry outside air, the pool felt refreshing. While floating
on my back and staring off into space, for a few magic moments I felt as
if a terrible weight had been lifted off my shoulders. If this chemo
continued to work, could Barry finally be rid of this illness, and could
our lives be back to normal? I could only hope so.

After our short visit to Texas, we returned to Urbana where we
finished out the school year. From late April through late May, Barry
had a hiatus from his chemotherapy. His doctors had suggested this in
order to minimize the toxicity of the drugs. So a few days after graduation, we drove up to Michigan for what had become our annual
weeklong end-of-school vacation. Our first stop was in Saugatuck, a
charming lakeside tourist town, and then on to Holland, where we
caught the yearly Tulip Festival. Photography has always been one of
my avocations, and these tulips provided ripe material. We spent hours
in the tulip fields while I captured the brilliant colors on film: first red,
then pink, then purple, orange, white, and even black. The two of us
posed before them as an older gentleman shot what would become our
annual holiday photo.

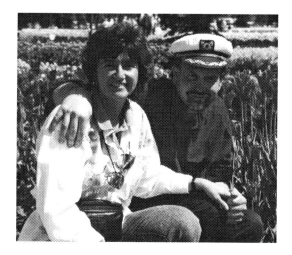

*At the tulip
festival posing
for our annual
holiday photo.
Holland,
Michigan; May
1995. (credit:
unknown)*

From Holland we drove north to another of our favorite spots, Michigan's "Little Finger," the northwest corner of the Lower Peninsula. We had discovered this region several years ago and its stunning scenery kept us coming back for more. It reminded us of California—minus the crowds and high prices. The marinas and the sailboats beckoned. I photographed Sleeping Bear Dunes National Lakeshore with its miles of sharp cliffs, white sandy beaches, and aquamarine waters. On one of our many hikes, I shot a photo of Barry walking along the dunes off into the sky. It looked as if he were at the end of the earth.

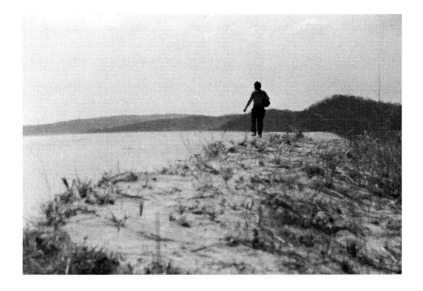

Barry hiking at Sleeping Bear Dunes National Lakeshore, Michigan; May 1995. (credit: author)

Barry resumed chemotherapy when we returned, completing his final regimen in late July 1995. On 4th of July weekend we drove to New England to visit my cousin, Jack, and his partner Steve. The three-day drive was rough on Barry, who was experiencing intense discomfort from diarrhea. In retrospect we would have been better off flying there. His stomach was on the blink during much of our stay, but that didn't stop him from being a tourist. One of our first stops was the Norman Rockwell Museum in Stockbridge, Massachusetts. Designed by architect Robert Stern, it had been featured in numerous architectural publications. Both Barry and I enjoyed Rockwell's artwork and we were fascinated by the museum. The paintings of "The Four Freedoms" impressed both of us. So did the simplicity of so many of his everyday American scenes, such as dinner around the Thanksgiving table. During the past year, I had come to appreciate settings like his all the more, and Rockwell's illustrations struck a chord with me. Barry, on the other hand, was most impressed by Rockwell's unsettling depictions of American racism.

Our final destination, Jack and Steve's house in rural Maine, was the perfect getaway spot. Their neo-Colonial home is set amidst over 60 acres of forest, clearing, bog, and meadow. Steve, a veterinarian, harbors many pets. During our visit their family included three horses, a rooster, a goat, two cats, and two charming Cairn Terriers. We fell in love with the small dogs, who escorted us everywhere we went. Jack and Steve and their friends took us on a boat ride through Portland Harbor, where we watched some magnificent 4th of July fireworks. Barry's stomach was feeling a bit unsettled on the boat but he still enjoyed the ride. Jack drove us up to spend a few days with my Aunt Georgia in Bangor. The four of us took a day trip to Campobello to visit the historic home of Franklin Delano Roosevelt, with its panoramic views of the Bay of Fundy.

Later that summer Barry and I embarked on a second Victory Tour of the San Francisco Bay Area. We also drove up to Ashland, Oregon, to visit other friends. Although it was a whirlwind tour, we managed to squeeze in our annual picnic at the Palace of Fine Arts. Reconnecting with our West Coast friends was a boost for both of us.

⸻

In the pre-dawn hours we flew from San Francisco to Houston for yet another visit to MD Anderson Cancer Center. In contrast to our visit there in May, this time the news was disappointing. Barry's latest CT-scan showed that the chemotherapy was no longer working. His body seemed to have developed a tolerance for 5-FU and interferon.

"We seem to have hit a brick wall," Dr. Curley said. "And at this point, I can safely say that the cancer will begin to grow again."

He advised discontinuing the chemotherapy until the cancer grew again in his liver. At that point Barry would have to go on MAID, a chemical cocktail that was highly toxic. While undergoing that treatment, Barry would have to stop working. MAID's side effects could include intense diarrhea, vomiting over a dozen times a day, and debilitating fatigue. Barry said he could handle it. But simply picturing him on that concoction made my own stomach begin to turn in knots.

Dr. Curley also notified us that Barry's hemoglobin level was only 9.7, and he recommended that Barry take iron supplements for a short while. Barry followed his advice.

Before we knew it, it was Labor Day weekend. I usually looked forward to long holiday weekends, but this one dragged like no other. Without warning, Barry collapsed and fainted while in the midst of a shower. Had it been only minutes later, I would have been off to our Saturday morning Farmer's Market at Urbana's Lincoln Square. Had it been later that day, we would have been driving up to Chicago to visit the renovated Navy Pier. And who knows what would have happened then? After hearing a loud thud, I ran into the bathroom and found him unconscious, lying in the bathtub. His skin was ashen, his body was limp, and his eyes were glazed over.

"Barry! Barry!" I shouted.

I grabbed him by the shoulders and shook him. But there was no response.

By now I thought that this was it, that he had just dropped dead in his tracks. My heart was beating so loudly that I could almost hear it. I quickly dialed 911. Minutes later, Barry miraculously came back to life.

"Don't panic!" I told him. "I just called 911, and an ambulance should be here any minute."

I quickly grabbed a towel, put it around him, and found his robe. Next I heard sirens howling and paramedics rushing towards our front door. They immediately administered oxygen to Barry and whisked him out of the house on a stretcher. I dashed into my car and followed the ambulance to the hospital. I was still trembling while I rushed to call Dr. Curley in Texas from the Emergency Room. For years, whenever I heard shower water running or a sudden, loud noise, I flashed back onto that scene. Hours later at the hospital, Barry's gastroenterologist, Dr. Lans, showed me an endoscopic photograph that he had just taken of Barry's stomach. After two years in hiding, the tumor had resurfaced. It was already five centimeters large. It turned out that the iron pills masked the fact that Barry had begun to bleed internally and his hemoglobin level had dropped to a precipitous 5.0. And also, despite his numerous CT-scans, his latest endoscopy was already eight months ago. None of his doctors had thought that test was medically necessary, especially while he was still on chemotherapy. Yet it was the endoscopy which could most easily detect tumor activity in the stomach. After this crisis was over, we insisted on an endoscopy every three months. No more emergencies, please!

Barry spoke with Dr. Curley later that day. The doctor suspected that a change in the biological behavior of the tumor had occurred, and that now it was a new ballgame. While his words usually reassured us, this time they did not. For the next several days, we waited in limbo while Barry was administered 11 blood transfusions. If his hemoglobin rose to 10, he could withstand this third operation. But if it didn't, there would be no operation, and that would be the end.

As had been the case two years ago, over 30 friends, neighbors, and colleagues stopped by to see Barry in the hospital. Several showered us both with cards, flowers, and small gifts.

While we were in this holding pattern, we met with Dr. X, one of the hospital's high-risk, re-operative surgeons. Barry had met him once before, as he had played a role in his first operation. But it was the first time I had seen him. Within just a few minutes, something about him rubbed me the wrong way.

"This operation is really serious. It's not like any other one you've had. That surgery you had in Texas—that wasn't a real operation! That one doesn't even count! You didn't even have to go down there for that. We could have done it right here," he informed us.

"Not according to what Dr. Johnson had told us months ago," we explained. "She said no one here was willing to do it."

"*I* could have. *I'm* the high-risk surgeon around here. You should have come to *me!*" he proclaimed.

But there was no point arguing with him.

Dr. X continued, "If we're lucky, we can remove the whole tumor. But if we're not, we may have to take the whole stomach with it. That would leave you having to eat out of a feeding tube. Are you ready for that? But first let's give you an MRI to see what it shows. And we need to compare it with your most recent CT-scan from MD Anderson. Your cancer may have grown so quickly between now and then that an operation isn't even possible. It could be socked in everywhere. It could be spreading like wildfire. If that's the case, then let's face it, *you're up shit creek without a paddle!*"

It was the first time I had heard this crass expression, and I never forgot it. His harsh words stuck with Barry and me like no others. We agreed that Dr. X had by far the worst bedside manner of any doctor we had ever seen. Too bad he was the only high-risk surgeon at our hospital. Weeks later, when Barry, Felicia, and I came in for a post-operative visit with Dr. X, he was equally surly.

"Sit down, Barry!" he ordered. "You know what your problem is? You just don't listen, that's what! You just don't listen! And you know what else? You're in denial—that's what!"

A medical intern stood dutifully at his side. I was tempted to find out his name and call him later to point out that Dr. X was about the worst role model he could find. As an educator myself, I was appalled. However, Barry and I held our tongues. It dawned on us that in our small college town, we might need Dr. X again someday.

While awaiting surgery, Barry kept himself busy by polishing up the finishing touches on his paper, "Into the Fever Swamps: The Radical Right Revisited," which he was scheduled to deliver at the Mid-America History Conference in Springfield, Missouri. It was an analysis of various far-right conspiracy theorists and prophets of doom, as well as the relationship between their values and that of society at large. Inspired by the 1995 Oklahoma City bombings, he was critical not only of the Radical Right, but also of its critics. The Mid-America conference was only a few days away, and now it was obvious that Barry would have to miss it. He was disappointed, as he had been a regular there for the past 10 years, and the only one he had skipped was when he was first stricken with cancer. So Barry called his colleague and friend, who found someone to read it for him.

In the meantime, I shuttled typewritten drafts of Barry's paper—with various hand-written notes scribbled along the margins—back and forth from his hospital bed to the nursing station. There a fax machine enabled the staff to shoot the paper down to Barry's departmental secretary in Charleston.

Barry had been admitted to the hospital on Saturday of Labor Day weekend, but it wasn't until the next Thursday that his operation actually took place. Our friend Diane took time off from work to join me in the vigil. Her gentle, soothing manner provided a sense of peace amidst all the chaos. We settled into our spot in the surgical waiting area, spreading out sandwiches, snacks, drinks, books, and musical tapes. By now I knew that being prepared could make the ordeal much less stressful. Hours later, as Diane sneaked out for a quick rest stop, a tall, thin man wearing a black shirt and a white collar walked into the room.

"Mrs. Riccio?" he called out.

"Yes," I responded as my eyes met his.

By now I had come to terms with the medical world, where I would always just be "Mrs. Riccio." But what did a minister want from me? Was the operation still in progress—or had something already gone wrong? Had Barry died on the operating table? Suddenly my legs felt weak and my face felt flushed.

"I just wanted to check in and see how you were doing," the minister replied as he sat down next to me, introduced himself, and shook my hand.

"What a relief!" I explained. "I thought something awful had happened."

I appreciated his visit, and we chatted for a bit, but I was definitely caught off guard. Minutes later, Diane reappeared at the doorway. With just one look at the minister and me, her mouth dropped. It took us both several minutes to recover.

After the operation was over, a volunteer aide told me that Dr. X was ready to meet with us. We had expected that surgery would last anywhere from 45 minutes to four hours, but only about an hour had passed.

"Let's go over to the private consultation room," he said.

I knew from experience what this meant.

"The operation was a success," he explained. "I was able to remove the tumor, and I had to cut out about one-third of his stomach. But I found little nodules around his pancreas, in his greater omentum, his belly cavity, and his lymph nodes. They're each about the size of the tip of my finger. The cancer is spreading all over the upper abdomen. And the liver is socked in. Don't even pretend that we're stopping it!

"There's no doubt in my mind that there will be a recurrence in a year. And then it could block the pancreas or the bowel. It's just a matter of time. It could be just months or even weeks. Barry's days are numbered. And as far as I'm concerned, he's still in total denial. He needs to set limits for what he can and can't do. It's spreading like wildfire."

I had tried to adhere to the old adage, "Hope for the best, but expect the worst." At least Barry's stomach was still intact, he did not need a feeding tube, and he could still enjoy eating. But the thought of the cancer roaring through him scared me. Once again my heart sank.

When Barry was wheeled back from the Recovery Room, he was suffering from a high fever. Diane found a wet wash cloth and routinely used it to wipe the sweat that was pouring off of Barry's forehead. So adept was she in her new role as a nurse that we later often referred to her as our Florence Nightingale. Once again I realized how lucky we both were to have such devoted friends.

While Barry was still hospitalized and recovering from surgery, his department chair, Anita, brought over a gift—an acclaimed book by a noted historian. He had also asked her to bring him his student papers so that he could begin grading them. A graduate student of his stopped by to visit, and Barry held an office hour from his hospital bed to discuss her thesis. He also had asked her to bring in her copy of the book, *Rotten Reviews*, and he asked me to bring in his yellow pad of paper.

For two hours during each of the three days following the operation, Barry, an avid reader of plays, wrote a play of his own. A steady stream of nurses paraded in and out of his room, checking his temperature, blood pressure, and pulse while Barry, pen in hand, immersed in thought, leaned over his yellow legal pad. He was still entangled in a maze of tubes but had somehow managed to free his right hand.

Barry had been carrying the ideas in his head for the past couple of years, and the little book, *Rotten Reviews*, served as a springboard. He had thought about writing a play for 20 years, after having been inspired by reading Arthur Miller's *All My Sons* while a sophomore in high school. He drew upon his own research into the world of the New York intellectuals, a group of largely Jewish and New York-based literary and social critics whose names were synonymous with American high-brow culture in the 1940's, 1950's, and 1960's. Barry's research on this subject found expression in a few conference papers and two articles, one of which won him the Carl Bode Award from the American Culture Association in 1994. Barry first learned of this award through a postcard sent to him by a friend. A few months later he received a formal letter of congratulations. Merely knowing that he had won a prize for his writing buoyed his spirits. As he put it at the time, "The dark cloud of cancer had been tempered by a ray of intellectual sunshine."

Scrawled out on his yellow legal pad was the first draft of his one-act play, *The Review.* In January 1997, the play would be produced at the Charleston Alley Theater. Here is how Barry described his play.

> It concerns the ethics of book reviewing, centering on the relationship between a New York literary critic and his literate wife, and the dilemma that he faced when *The New York Times* asked him to write a review of his one-time mentor's latest collection of essays. The play is a commentary on the nature of criticism and the tension between the loyalties that we have to the truth and those that we have to each other. It features a great deal of witty repartee, but it also has an edge. It is no mere drawing-room comedy.

Two weeks later Barry returned home. Under ordinary circumstances a patient just released from the hospital would prefer to spend his first evening resting at home, but not so in Barry's case. Two friends of ours had invited us over for dinner that evening, so together we celebrated his great escape. Barry's stomach was still sore from the operation so he couldn't fully appreciate the meal, but he loved the company. And for several days more, he had to eat mainly soft foods and small meals, something that did not come easily to him. But eventually his stomach healed, and within a few weeks he was back teaching.

My 40th birthday fell on September 11, 1995, when Barry was still hospitalized. The night before, three friends had taken me out for dinner at one of my favorite restaurants. I held up fine through the dinner and was energized by their company. But when I woke up the next morning on my big day, I couldn't help but feel sorry for myself. Over the years we had been to numerous surprise parties for friends of ours who had hit the big 4-0. Not that I expected one myself, but spending most of the day at Carle Hospital was not exactly what I had in mind. Normally I would have spent the day working at the Building Research Council. But keenly aware that I was emotionally fragile, and having no classes to teach that day, I had planned to take the day off. I was afraid that I might burst into tears if someone decided to throw a birthday party for me at work. I didn't even want to take that chance. I could plug my finger in the dike for just so long.

That morning I went for a swim at my favorite indoor pool. Afterwards I felt refreshed and ready to face the day. When I returned home, the phone started ringing. Several family members from both coasts called to wish me a happy birthday. And I received cards from every relative I had. I was especially touched by three care packages that arrived from my parents, my sister, and my sister-in-law. Under these circumstances, I needed all the TLC I could get. I spent the rest of the morning and afternoon in the hospital with Barry.

That evening, I had arranged to meet some of my friends at a local Chinese restaurant where our women faculty in environmental design had been getting together for years. Up until the last minute, I wasn't sure if I felt up to going. I didn't even know if I could muster up enough energy to make it from the house to my car. But that afternoon, my friend Sharon called to ask if I wanted a ride. And that made my decision for me. When we walked into the dining room, about 10 friends were waiting for me at our regular table with cards, gifts, and beautiful bouquets of flowers. And despite my feeling blue earlier that day, I had a great time. Once again I was rescued.

———•—•———

Our fifth and final trip to Texas was in October 1995. My cousin, Andoni, who lived in Dallas, flew in to have lunch with us just before our doctor's appointment.

"Be strong, both of you," he advised us. "You have always been strong. I can't imagine what it must feel like to be in your shoes."

His words echoed in our minds later that day when we received even more devastating news. It was October 11, a date we'll never forget. By now even our experts at MD Anderson Cancer Center had

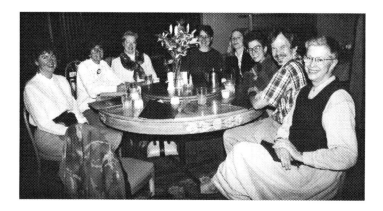

Barry was in the hospital recuperating from his third cancer operation while friends treated me for my 40th birthday. I was so drained that I almost didn't make it to my own party. L–R: Anne Marshall, myself, Barb Selby, Lisa Busjahn, Kate Brown, Sharon Irish, Jory Johnson, Eliza Steelwater. Champaign, Illinois; September 1995. (credit: Robert Selby)

run out of options. After reviewing the latest set of CT-scans and other chemosensitivity tests on Barry's recent stomach tumor, Dr. Curley concluded that no further treatment would work. Even the prospect of MAID, the powerful form of chemotherapy that he had suggested earlier, was now out. It was not worth the highly toxic side effects. Of course, Barry could try one or two courses just to see what would happen. Or he could try some other forms of chemotherapy, but all others that he could think of simply were not worth the risk. Barry's liver could fail. His kidney could fail. And he could die from the chemotherapy itself. Barry then asked him the key question.

"Given all this, how much time do you think I have left?"

The doctor hesitated to answer.

"I have a couple patients with multiple spots and the same kind of biological change as you who have lived three to four years. But I've seen others live only a year or less. If it continues to grow at this point, it could be only two to four months before you start feeling symptoms. Or you might not feel any pain for another year, or even 16 months. It depends how fast the cancer grows. The cancer in your belly cavity could kill you before the cancer in the liver.

"Barry, sometimes we can't cure all our patients."

As Barry later recalled, "I thought to myself, this is not the point, whether or not I can be cured. I wasn't going to MD Anderson for a cure anyway. I was going there to keep on living."

"What would you do if you were in my shoes?" Barry asked the doctor.

Barry's face was flushed, and he was beginning to feel hot.

Again the doctor wavered.

"I would want to feel as well as possible for as long as possible. Quality of life concerns would be most important to me now," he replied.

In just minutes, the wind had been knocked out of our sails. We were both devastated. This time my emotions got the best of me, and for a few hours, even Barry was taken aback. After leaving Dr. Curley's office, we both felt dazed as we made our way through the corridors.

"Let's go see Sister Alice," I said. "I think we both need someone to talk to right now."

"You're right. Let's go," Barry said.

We sought the counsel of Sister Alice, whom we had met during her cancer support groups. We tracked her down at her shoebox-size office tucked away in the basement of the hospital. Sister Alice listened carefully. Watching the tears stream down my cheeks, she handed me some tissues. She also offered us some advice.

"Enjoy the time you have together. You never know what may happen in the meantime. Something just might come through for you."

In an attempt to lift us out of our funereal mood that evening, we took the Rotary House shuttle over to Rice Village. After our many visits to Houston, the Village had become our Great Escape. To us, this district—with its trendy eateries, chic boutiques, and bright lights—had always looked so upbeat. But this time all the flashy sights and sounds seemed to blur together. Even our taste buds seemed to have gone dead. We could barely swallow our dinners. We meandered around the neighborhood, venturing in and out of a few shops. At the time I thought that being in a public place was better than heading back to our hotel room to brood over this latest bombshell.

"So how are *you* two doing tonight?" chirped the saleswomen.

"Do you *really* want to know?" I said to myself. "How about telling them, 'This was the worst day of my entire life! How would you feel if your husband were just given a death sentence?'"

But instead Barry and I glanced at each other as we blurted out a barely audible "o.k."

We walked and walked, talked and talked, circling block after block. The day's news kept playing over and over again in our heads like a nasty tape recording. Dr. Curley and MD Anderson had been our lifeline for the past year. If one of the world's top cancer centers had now run out of options, what were we to do? Were we back to square one? What next? What was to become of us?

"I'm not ready to become a widow!" I lamented. "I'm too young! And, Barry, you're too young to have to go through this!"

That evening we borrowed a video from the Rotary House's Laughter Library, a comedy entitled *It Could Happen to You.* A nice try, but it was impossible to take our minds off our own melodrama that had played out that day. The next morning we checked out of Rotary House well before the crack of dawn. As my eyes scanned our peach-colored hotel room one last time, I realized that we would never again see this lovely place. For the past year it had become our lifeboat. My eyes were raw and swollen from crying all night long. I barely slept a wink. Inserting my contact lenses was impossible, so I didn't even try. I could barely see as we plugged along on our monotonous three-hour drive from the St. Louis Airport to Champaign in time for my 4:00 seminar.

When we finally arrived home, I had only 15 minutes to race inside, change my clothes, use the bathroom, and hurry back to school. In an attempt to hide from any colleagues who might ask about my trip, I sneaked up the back stairway of the Architecture Building to my class in room 210A. Even an innocent, "Well, how are you doing, Kathy?" might have put me over the edge. I camouflaged my eyes with glasses, hoping that my students would not notice the terrible shape I was in. I still wonder how I managed to teach my class that day. But I had already missed so many days of work that I didn't want to miss one more.

A machine gun was aiming right at us, and it just wouldn't stop firing. Could we keep dodging bullets, and just how much more could we take? Could we possibly gear up enough energy to start all over again, and where else could we go? Could we still find a cure—or was it already too late? Our Lone Star Journeys were over. We simply had no choice. Now we were forced to pursue more options on our own. Barry put it well.

The one institution that was providing us with hope—the one institution that was comforting, nurturing, and reassuring—the one institution that was on the cutting edge of scientific research—had now given up on me. To be sure, I would be monitored and my pain would be attended to. But there were no other measures to be taken. In sum, MD Anderson had raised the white flag. They had surrendered, but I had not yet begun to fight.

CHAPTER THREE

Buying Time
(1995-1996)

"ONE COOL JUDGEMENT IS WORTH A THOUSAND HASTY COUNCILS."
—WOODROW WILSON

From day one, we had always been open about our plight. Virtually anyone who knew us was aware of Barry's cancer. Friends from across the country suggested many different avenues of treatment for us to pursue, and we discussed each with our local oncologist and with Dr. Curley. Ironically, one of the best ideas came from our neighbors Carole and Tino, only two doors away.

This couple had been intimately involved with our case from the beginning, as it was at their home just two years ago that Barry had collapsed. Carole and Tino informed us about photodynamic light therapy, an innovative technique used in the plant and animal world that is occasionally applied to humans. It involves shining strong, concentrated beams of laser lights on cancerous growths that would otherwise be invisible. Ideally, it could prevent cancer from recurring or spreading any further. Tino had conducted photodynamic light therapy on plants.

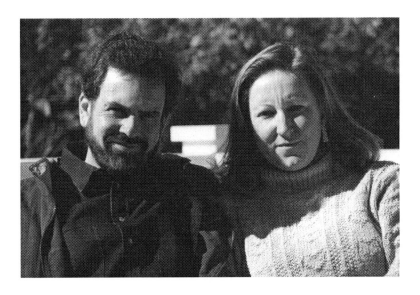

Just days after we received the devastating news in Texas that no more could be done to control Barry's cancer, our friend Colleen Casey flew out from San Francisco to visit us. She was just what the doctor ordered. Urbana, Illinois: October 1995. (credit: author)

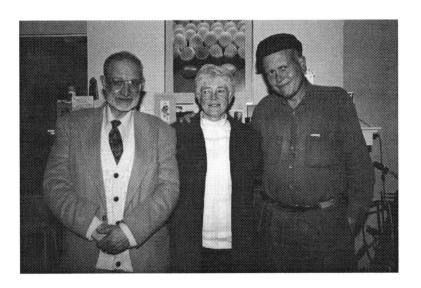

A later shot of Barry with our long time neighbors and friends, Carole and Tino Rebeiz. It was at their house that Barry first collapsed. Without them, we would never have known about photodynamic light therapy, the procedure Barry underwent at the Detroit Medical Center. Urbana, Illinois: October 1999. (credit: author)

According to our neighbors, one of the leading researchers about photodynamic light therapy was located in Canada, and they gave Barry his contact information. Shortly after that, Barry called him up to find out whether or not he was beginning to apply this research on humans. He was not.

However, the researcher explained, "Some studies are being conducted in England. And I am aware of only one such application in the US: by a Dr. David Fromm at the Detroit Medical Center. Perhaps Dr. Fromm could help you."

No sooner did Barry get off the phone to Canada than he got on the phone to Michigan. After hearing about Barry's dilemma, Dr. Fromm sounded intrigued by his case. He and Barry connected instantly. He gave Barry all his telephone numbers, including one at his home, and encouraged him to call any time. Never had we seen any of our doctors do this for us before. He was the first of our doctors to have e-mail, and on occasion we contacted him that way. He always responded immediately.

After looking up his entry in *Who's Who in America*, we found that he was Surgeon in Chief at Detroit Medical Center, part of Wayne State University. And we also learned that at age 38, while at Syracuse, he had been the youngest Chief of Surgery in the entire country. Not only was Dr. Fromm unusually accessible, but he was also extremely renowned in his field. We were definitely starting off on the right foot.

Within hours I copied off Barry's relevant medical records —all his operative reports, pathology reports, and his latest CT-scan results — and faxed them away to Dr. Fromm. After reviewing Barry's case, he informed us that he could indeed try to remove the cancer from Barry's greater omentum and belly cavity using photodynamic light therapy. It appeared that while other doctors had all but given up on Barry, this energetic surgeon had come to our rescue.

In the meantime, we discussed the possibility of this upcoming operation with Dr. Johnson, and we also checked in with Dr. Curley. Neither discouraged us from proceeding. Over the years we had gotten in the habit of reviewing with both doctors various treatment alternatives. For instance, Barry was taking shark cartilage pills. While neither doctor recommended them, neither panned the practice. Ditto for Essiac, the tea-like substance that was supposed to shrink tumors. Barry had been drinking that for several months as well. For a while they seemed to be having a positive effect, yet eventually his cancer continued to grow and he discontinued both of them. He was also taking a slew of vitamins and supplements, including B, C, E, potassium, selenium, echinacea, and garlic.

More often than not, the doctors' response was, "There's no scientific evidence that any of these help cancer patients. But there's also no evidence that they hurt. So go ahead and take them if you like."

We also discussed several other alternatives that well-meaning friends had mentioned. In most cases, both doctors warned us to beware of several approaches that raised red flags. One involved a doctor in Texas who claimed to cure cancer patients through a regular series of treatments in his office. I contacted him, requesting the names of leiomyosarcoma patients who had been cured by his approach. His assistant could only offer the name of one woman, and her cancer was in a different site from Barry's. But just one patient was not enough for me. It was beginning to sound shady. But when we read through his brochure and learned that the price tag just to initiate the treatment was $100,000, we knew something was amiss. For one, we didn't have anywhere near that kind of money. Neither do most people. For another, we both believed that taking advantage of patients in their most desperate hour was clearly vile. When we ran all this by Dr. Johnson, she informed us that the journals in which this doctor had published were suspect. Even worse, he refused to share his findings with the scientific community. And he had no statistics upon which patients could rely. Dr. Curley's assessment was similar. In short, both our doctors believed him to be a shyster. Months later when we saw the same doctor featured on ABC's "Nightline" because of a 75-count indictment by the federal government, we felt vindicated.

Yet another of these questionable treatment programs was in Mexico. We learned of this facility through a contact on the Internet and sent away for literature. But, again, our doctors steered us away, informing us that after going there for treatment, several patients had died. So when Dr. Johnson and Dr. Curley sanctioned photodynamic light therapy, we felt relieved.

Nonetheless, the prospect of going to Detroit scared me. I feared the unknown. Although initially I had felt anxious about going to

Houston, the place soon grew on me. Traveling there from the Midwest in the dead of winter, it was a treat to see green grass and flowers in bloom. And after five visits to Houston, I knew what to expect. But this trip was different. As the day of our departure drew near, the more my stomach was tied up in knots. While I knew that it could be a boon for Barry medically, deep in my heart I dreaded going.

Here is what Barry was feeling at the time.

> I felt nervous for a few weeks before going to Detroit. But I felt reassured by the doctor and his willingness to try what no other doctor was willing to try on me.
>
> I took small comfort in the fact that no matter how much pain and fear I would feel in the hospital, much of it would be tempered by the drugs I would be on. One of those drugs —morphine, in particular —if anything, generally put patients in a fairly good mood. Also, I was exceedingly eager to meet the doctor with whom I had spoken over the phone so many times. He seemed highly intelligent, articulate, and personable. Just before we left there was an undercurrent of anxiety running through me. It was not unusual for me to have those sorts of feelings on the verge of any watershed experience.

So in this third phase of our medical odyssey, the Motor City became our medical Mecca. Just days after a Thanksgiving dinner with friends, we sped off our holiday letters, finished our classes early, packed our bags, and left home. The mad rush reminded me of our departure for Houston just a year before. I hadn't even had time to buy one Christmas present.

As we drove towards the medical center, it took us only a few seconds to realize that the surrounding neighborhood was deadly. In fact, it was one of the most depressing places either of us had ever seen. Indeed, it resembled New York City's South Bronx and Chicago's South Side. As we gazed out our car window, we rode by blocks and blocks of what looked like bombed-out, abandoned apartment buildings. Row upon row of windows were broken or missing, front doors were boarded up, and streets and sidewalks were strewn with litter. An occasional human being or two surfaced, but most appeared to be drug addicts, homeless, or other members of the down-and-out. It looked like a virtual war zone. We could also see that we had absolutely no place to walk except for the medical center itself, which included Harper Hospital, a Children's Hospital and a Veteran's Hospital. Only two eateries were within walking distance, and both were at Harper Hospital: a cafeteria and a Wendy's.

Both our mothers joined us for Barry's hospital stay, leaving their homes in the sunny Southwest to be at our sides in the dead of the midwestern winter. My mother, Anne, came from La Jolla and Felicia from Scottsdale —both a far cry from Detroit.

The International Center/Guest Housing was a high-rise apartment building set up to accommodate patients' families, outpatients, and medical interns and residents. Its lobby and corridors emitted the musty, unpleasant odor of a nursing home. Walking down the hallways we whiffed an unappealing mixture of cooking fumes and Ajax cleanser. A diminutive plastic Christmas tree was prominently displayed in the lobby, a far cry from the lavish display at the Rotary House. Decorated with a handful of token ornaments, it provided a faint attempt at some holiday cheer. With only one exception, the staff at the desk were curt and abrupt. Public relations were not their forte. Even worse, after 8:00 p.m. every weeknight, after 4:00 p.m. on Saturday and all day Sunday, the lobby desk sat empty. Every time I parked the car, I did a 360-degree check before unlocking the doors to make sure no one was waiting to jump us. Then we walked quickly to the front door, through the lobby and into the elevator. Only when I locked myself in our apartment did I feel safe. I couldn't figure out how I could possibly last two weeks in this horrible place.

Whenever we visited Barry in the hospital after dark, we needed to call a security escort. About 20 minutes later a van arrived to pick us up, and the driver steered us around a long block to the main entrance even though by day, it was only a few yards away. A few times we struck up a conversation with the driver.

Once he told us, "Don't worry, ladies! This neighborhood may look pretty bad to you now, but it's much safer now than it was years ago. You should have seen it before! Now everyone has moved out, and there is no one left to mug!"

He meant to reassure us, but his words were cold comfort.

We were not the only ones to find the environment unsettling. Crime seemed to be on the minds of many Guest Housing residents. Whenever we saw human beings walk down the hallway and into their rooms, the sound of the deadbolt instantly followed. One evening Barry and I escorted his mother to her room, as she was afraid to go there alone.

> The key to her room didn't seem to fit very easily that night. I turned it a few times, and couldn't figure out why it wasn't working this time. I felt that something was amiss. But I was able to push open the door, because apparently it hadn't been locked in the first place. Much to my amazement, I discovered a Middle Eastern woman, her head wrapped up in a Chodor, with a look of horror on her face —her three startled children were no less terrified. The room was dark and smelled of incense. Religious symbols lined the walls. Clearly this was not my mother's room. I apologized profusely and closed the door at once. Luckily her husband was not at home. In fact, we were on the wrong floor. A wave of hysteria engulfed us, and for 10 minutes, we just couldn't stop laughing. It was the first time any of us had been mistaken for a criminal.

The apartment that Mom and I shared was actually not bad. Ironically, at $67 a night, it proved to be nearly as expensive as Rotary House. It was a one-bedroom unit with a foldout couch in the living room near the TV. She slept on the couch while I used the queen-sized bed. Two windows in the living room and the bedroom were large enough to get a good view of the parking lot, the treetops, and the city in the distance. The most pleasant part of our vista was watching parents drop off their children at the medical center employees' day care center located on the first floor of our building. The kids were all bundled up in colorful snowsuits, hats, scarves, and mittens. Sometimes, even from our room several stories high, we could hear them laughing. It was a welcome sound.

I was especially pleased that Mom was able to make the trip, and I was looking forward to spending time with her. She and I made great roommates. Given that we normally saw each other for only a few days a year, it was a welcome opportunity to reconnect. I always enjoyed her company. Never losing her cool, she would help diffuse the tension and put me at ease. She was a good sport, willing to go anywhere I wanted, and always easily entertained in a shopping mall or a lively downtown. Like me, she was content to play tourist when we had some spare moments away from the hospital. But Mom was also willing to work. She and I made several runs to the nearest grocery store, Farmer Jack's, to stock up on food and household supplies. There we were among the few non-African-Americans to be found. Although she was not used to being a racial minority herself, this didn't faze her at all. While I felt slightly uncomfortable at first, it made me realize how persons of color must feel every day in an all-white environment. Mom and I routinely lugged the grocery bags up to our apartment and filed away all the items into our refrigerator. Nor did she mind cooking regularly for all four of us. The aromas of oven-baked chicken soon filled the apartment, and it began to smell like home. With Mom in the kitchen, we ate well.

Harper Hospital harked back to the Civil War era, though it was hardly charming. In fact, much of it looked as if it were out of a Dickens novel —cold, gray, and grim. Like most hospitals, it was built in stages. Navigating through it was like finding one's way through a labyrinth. Its massive exterior walls were a dirty, dark brick; victims of Detroit's harsh climate and years of soot and pollution. At night, with the fluorescent lights glowing through the windows, the place looked downright spooky. Its interior walls were virtually barren and the lighting was reminiscent of those squalid detective stations from old movie melodramas.

As Barry put it,

> It reminded me of the asylum in which Olivia de Havilland was incarcerated in the famous 1940's film, *The Snake Pit.*

Based on what we had heard, we expected Detroit to have a horrid downtown. And we were not let down. Few people were on the street by day, and by night virtually no one was around. We drove through the city center several times hoping to find at least one place that would lure us out of the car, but not much luck. While Barry was in the hospital, Mom, Felicia, and I visited the infamous Renaissance Center where I could see firsthand that my late colleague William Whyte's harsh criticism of it was well deserved. It was one of the most uninviting spaces I have ever seen —a fortress perched high above the rest of the city, its glimmering glass towers surrounded by a maze of concrete parking garages.

Nonetheless both before and after Barry's operation, we all kept ourselves entertained by discovering the pleasures of Greektown, just a few miles away. There I devoured my avgolemono soup and pastitso and moussaka. When I closed my eyes it almost felt like being at home.

Another of Detroit's bright spots was the Motown Museum, which the four of us visited soon after Barry's release from the hospital. Listening to the rapid rhythm of The Temptations, The Supremes, and The Four Tops perked me up. And I was fascinated by their costume displays, ablaze with color and sparkling sequins.

We also discovered Birmingham and Grosse Point, two aristocratic suburbs. While I had heard of the latter, I had never heard of the former. But what a place! Birmingham's festive decor put us in the holiday spirit. Lights were flashing everywhere, handsome displays were shining in every store window, and Christmas carols were streaming from speakers hidden in the trees. Despite the gray skies and temperatures in the teens, simply walking the downtown streets was uplifting. Unlike Detroit, its sidewalks were full of people day and night. It had a real, old-fashioned downtown. As a result, we made the half-hour drive out to Birmingham a few times. Like Rice Village, it had become our Great Escape. Mom, who grew up in Maine, relished the winter weather. She delighted in bundling up in her scarf, hat, and gloves. At times I hardly recognized this Southern Californian.

Fortunately, Dr. Fromm performed surgery on Barry's greater omentum, removing it and the cancer with it. He also removed the cancer from Barry's belly cavity. The operation was a success. Dr. Fromm did not "go all the way" with his novel light therapy procedure. He shone some light on the subject, but he did not use the special infrared light that would have carried photodynamic light therapy to completion. He said he did not need to go further because he was able to remove the problems surgically. Barry reflected on this latest turn of events.

At the very least I was relieved, for just before the operation Dr. Fromm had me feel precisely where the cancer was in my abdomen. I had never actually felt any tumor activity there before. The liver, of course, was another matter. Dr. Fromm indicated to me that he would tackle that problem in the late spring, after my semester was over.

By this point, I was unaccustomed to good news. So this time it felt even better. Despite the bleak surroundings, our trip had been worthwhile. To top it off, while making his rounds, at Barry's request, Dr. Fromm even brought him a cup of tea.

The doctor was terrific, and his interns and residents were very competent. After completing Barry's operation and finding the three of us in the waiting area, he drew a diagram on a chalkboard explaining exactly what had just happened. He spent several minutes with us, and answered every one of our questions. In this respect, he reminded me of Dr. Curley. I felt fortunate to have found such good medical care.

Success came at a price. For 48 grueling hours after surgery, Barry was forced to wear oversized sunglasses —the kind skiers wear — wrapped halfway around his head. His eyes were totally hidden from view, as the procedure had made them unusually sensitive to light. When I first saw him after the operation, he was lying in his bed, wearing those odd-looking shades. He reminded me of Alfredo, the Italian movie projectionist in the film, *Cinema Paradiso,* who became blind after his theater was burned to the ground. Even though it was still light outside, Barry's hospital room was pitch dark. The depressing green and yellow print curtains were taped shut with several strips of ugly gray adhesive. All light switches were taped "Off." Only a faint light was glowing ever so slightly from underneath his bed. It was by far the most macabre of all our hospital scenes. To me, it felt as if he were completely cut off from the outside world. Yet for Barry, it was far worse.

Recuperating in Harper Hospital wasn't quite like the postoperative experience I had at MD Anderson. For one, I wasn't allowed to take any Tylenol after the inevitable fever developed. The medical staff informed me that Tylenol only masked the symptoms. For another, I had to wear this curious "shield," as the doctors called it. Supposedly this device made one cough more effectively. Unfortunately my coughs were not particularly effective, though they were painful.

With one exception, the nursing staff was mediocre and not particularly friendly. They didn't smile much, they didn't display much energy, and they hardly talked at all. Nor did they seem to know that much whenever I asked them questions. They didn't volunteer much information, nor did they seem all that interested in how I actually felt. To me they acted as if they were merely doing a job, as if they were there to complete their shift. They would do whatever was minimally necessary and only that. They didn't go an extra inch. This was in sharp contrast to the nursing staff at Carle Hospital as well as at MD Anderson. While I would give those nurses an "A," the ones in Detroit would get a "C" at best. They simply did what they had to do to get by.

But the pain was a relatively minor problem. What perhaps bothered me most was having to wear those big, thick sunglasses for at least 48 hours. I didn't much like the looks of the place to begin with, but barely being able to see anything did not help matters any. That was bad enough, but what made the situation even more eerie was that not a single light could be turned on in my room during that entire period. Even the shades had to be drawn. And, needless to say, I couldn't leave the room, read a magazine, or watch television. I could take phone calls, however, and luckily I did have a fair number. When I was finally able to "see the light," I immediately devoured an issue of Newsweek and quickly began to catch up on my Cable news programs.

Here, too, we received scores of get-well wishes, flowers, and holiday letters from our family and friends around the world. With each one, our spirits were buoyed. For me, just like the year before in Texas, checking our mailbox was one of the highlights of the day. And even though we didn't know a soul in the city of Detroit, we did have two visitors who came to see us after Barry shed his sunglasses. One of them had been one of Barry's favorite students at Eastern Illinois University. She and her husband arrived with a small poinsettia plant wrapped up in gold foil with a red bow. It decorated Barry's hospital room and became our symbolic Christmas tree. It lasted through the long plane ride out to California, where it made its way to my parents' house. Years later, miraculously, it survived. Mom believed that as long as Barry was alive, the poinsettia, too, would hang on. In fact, he outlasted it.

Every day I had been anxiously checking the weather forecast on TV, fearing that a blizzard would leave us stranded in Detroit through the Christmas holidays. It was not our favorite city. But the weather cooperated, and the snow never arrived. On Christmas Eve we crammed ourselves onto a full flight and escaped to California.

Barry was still in his postsurgical recovery, and he was not allowed to lift more than six pounds. He carried a small knapsack with him, and the rest of his luggage was checked. Per doctor's orders, we transported him through the Detroit Airport in a wheelchair, which, despite his protestations, allowed us to maneuver around the holiday crowds. Everywhere we turned, we collided with bulging suitcases, overflowing shopping bags, and brightly wrapped Christmas presents. At every gate, wall to wall bodies filled row after row of black vinyl seats, spilling out onto the floor. If one could pick an ideal day of the year for air travel, Christmas Eve would not be it.

Inching my way down the aisle, I managed to squeeze into my pint-sized airplane seat. My face was glued to the window as we sped down the runway and bolted into the sky. Soaring above the clouds, the Detroit suburbs came into view. As we reached our cruising altitude, I turned up the volume on my CD. Pianist Hilton Ruiz was playing my favorite version of "Santa Claus is Coming to Town." I sensed an uncontrollable smile forming. A few stray tears welled up in my eyes, blurring the scenery below. The more we climbed, the more I felt the heavy load of the past few weeks began to lighten.

Barry, a political news junkie, spent most of the flight catching up on his newspapers and magazines. While held captive in the hospital, he had fallen behind on current events. Even though his painkillers made him drowsy, he managed to stay awake all the way to the West Coast.

"I was glad Detroit was behind me. I was glad the operation was a success. And I was looking forward to going to California," he said. At St. Louis, our foursome went our separate ways. Felicia flew home to Phoenix, and the three of us continued out to the Golden State.

Hours later we made our dramatic descent into San Diego. Off to our left were the skyscrapers of downtown, and off to our right, the magnificent buildings of Balboa Park. The California sun was shining. The bay was glistening. Sailboats danced along the waters. As we dipped even further, rows of palm trees swayed in the breeze. Bam! The wheels hit the runway! Mom and I started clapping.

"We made it!" we both shouted.

"Welcome to San Diego," announced the flight attendant. "And Merry Christmas to all of you!"

Not only had we arrived on the other side of the country. We had landed on another planet.

As we climbed up the steep tunnel, I could see Dad standing in the doorway. He was at his usual spot at the head of the line. His arms were outstretched, his eyes opened wide, and a giant smile was on his face.

"Welcome! Welcome!" he shouted.

In fact, life as a temporary bachelor had not suited him at all. After being separated from Mom for two long weeks, and despite having called us every day, he had been miserable. But when he saw all three of us he lit up.

After the short ride along I-5 up to La Jolla, we settled into my parents' guestroom. Even though the sun was streaming in, Barry could hardly keep his eyes open.

After an all-too-short nap, we woke up in time to attend Christmas Eve services at my parents' church in Cardiff-by-the-Sea. The next day we drove up to Irvine and had a festive Christmas dinner with my sister Mary Anne, and brother-in-law, John, and their family. John's mother, who had been diagnosed with cancer earlier that year, was living with them at the time.

As we all bowed our heads in prayer before the meal, John said, "We have lots to be thankful about this Christmas. We are grateful, Mom, that you are still with us. And we are grateful, Barry, that you are still with us, and that you could travel to be with us after your operation. Thanks, God, for being so good to our family."

We raised our glasses in a toast, "Good health to us all for the New Year!"

Between Christmas and New Year's, Barry made the one-hour flight to Phoenix to spend some time with his family. Over the holiday break, Barry regained his strength. When he returned to La Jolla, he and I resumed our walking routine. During one warm, sunny day, we hiked several miles along the steep cliffs of Coast Walk, down past the La Jolla Cove, the Children's Pool, and all the way to Windansea, the famous surfing beach. Anyone who saw Barry would never know that only weeks ago he had been under the knife.

———————

In January we returned home. By now we had been gone almost a month, and it felt good to be back. Indeed, settling back into our daily routines was comforting; we had reached the point where we craved normality. How I wished that whenever someone would call us, we could simply report, "We're just fine. Nothing is new."

But no, something new was always happening on the medical scene, and we had way too much to tell. Barry never hesitated to give a point-by-point account to anyone. He could easily spend an hour engrossed in a phone conversation and as soon as he hung up and the phone rang once more, do it all over again. Sometimes it seemed that our entire Saturday and Sunday mornings were spent talking on the phone. On the other hand, I felt that I had seen, heard, and been through enough to last a lifetime. The last thing in the world I wanted to do was talk about it. It was like scraping an old wound over and over again. I just wanted to leave it alone. I yearned to focus on the present and not to rehash the past. On occasion I purposely slipped out early to run my Saturday morning errands just so that I would miss the barrage of phone calls.

At work, I was constantly accosted by well-meaning colleagues who would ask, "How's Barry?" whenever they saw me. Several stopped me in my tracks, no matter how fast I was walking, no matter how heavy a load of books I was carrying, no matter how hard I tried to avoid their gaze. Over the years I had developed two sets of responses, a more informative one for those whom we knew well, and a Readers' Digest condensed version for those whom we did not. Although I appreciated their concern, and I always ended my remarks with "Thank you for asking," in retrospect this may have been a mistake. It only encouraged further questioning. The never-ending inquiries often made me feel as if my primary identity was now as the wife of a sick man. I wanted to be perceived as the person I always was, not as Florence Nightingale.

I had always been fairly private at work, keeping my personal life to myself as much as possible. And yet once Barry's illness became known, I felt as if our living room door had blown wide open. Any semblance of privacy was now gone. Every last detail of his illness became public knowledge. I felt as if I had a scarlet letter, a huge "C" engraved on my forehead that branded me for years. No matter how hard I tried to wash it off it was still there for all to see.

In many ways, dealing with cancer day-to-day had given us a new perspective on several aspects of life. For example, at times we were both struck by those individuals we knew who, no matter what, always seemed to complain. In fact, academia seems to breed whiners. In response to our usual "How are you?" their answers were always the same.

"I'm swamped! I'm so busy! I don't know how I can handle it!"

"You just can't imagine all that I have to do by the end of this week. It's making me crazy!"

"Life is just awful. The stress is getting to me!"

Secretly Barry and I would both smile. They really thought they had it bad. Although we didn't discount their own travails, we couldn't help but wonder how they could possibly handle a situation like ours.

Still others we knew elsewhere were in a constant quest for something: a more luxurious home, a more expensive car, or a higher-paying job. No matter what they already had, they were always seeking more. I began to feel sorry for people like this. Little did they realize how fortunate they were to have the most prized possessions of all: good health and the love of those around them. Happiness was already in their grasp, if they would only redefine it.

Between work schedules, often in the early evenings, we sandwiched in our walks. Sundays were a ritual. From about 9:00 on, "Reliable Sources," "This Week with David Brinkley", and other morning news shows kept us transfixed. When the talking heads had finished, we walked the tree-lined streets of our neighborhood to The Corner Store to pick up *The New York Times*. The owner always set aside a copy for us, and if no other customers were around, he would stop to chat. A bespectacled man with gray hair and a low-key demeanor, he epitomized Urbana's friendly, small-town feel. His tiny store at the edge of campus was the only one of its kind, offering a variety of snacks, sundries, and medicines. It was a welcome antidote to the giant WalMart and Meijer superstores that had invaded the north edge of Champaign-Urbana. Two years later, when I drove by the corner of Lincoln and Nevada and discovered that The Corner Store was no more, I felt a pang of nostalgia.

The Corner Store was only about a mile from home, so if we felt energetic enough, we kept walking even further west towards campus. The U of I quad with its grand Georgian buildings beckoned. Shrouded in snow, it was a winter wonderland. In springtime, when the saucer magnolia, dogwood, and cherry trees were in full bloom, an explosion of pink and white. In summer, with its lush, dark green foliage and steam rising from the pavement, a sultry scene from the South. In fall, an artist's palette of orange, yellow, and red. We always found a visit there uplifting.

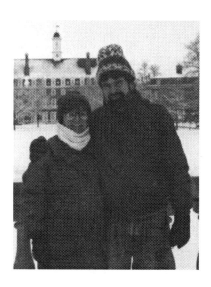

At the University of Illinois quad, a winter wonderland and a popular destination for our weekend walks. Urbana, Illinois; February 1994. (credit: unknown)

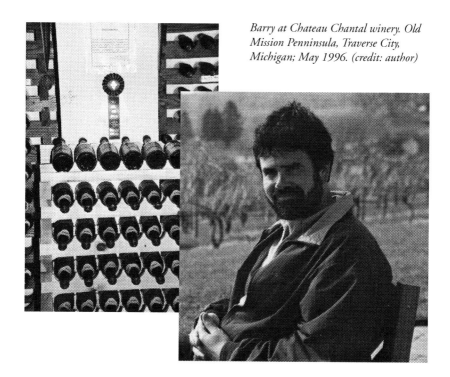

Barry at Chateau Chantal winery. Old Mission Penninsula, Traverse City, Michigan; May 1996. (credit: author)

We walked even more that May during our annual vacation in western Michigan. Once again we returned to photograph Holland's tulip fields and hike at Sleeping Bear Dunes. As it had always done in the past, the magnificent scenery boosted our spirits.

———◆———

In early June 1996, we drove off to Michigan once again. Despite the fact that a year and a half earlier, Dr. Curley had concluded that an operation on Barry's liver could not remove all the cancer, Dr. Fromm was willing to give it another try. Given Dr. Fromm's success rescuing the cancer from Barry's belly cavity only months before, we were hopeful that he could be our lifeboat once more. Just as we had felt so reassured to have Barry in the hands of Dr. Curley at MD Anderson, we felt equally optimistic to have him under the care of Dr. Fromm.

For weeks, as I ticked off the dates in my calendar getting closer and closer to the month of June, I dreaded the thought of going back there. Just thinking about it made my stomach turn in knots. Although I was grateful that Dr. Fromm was willing to take the risk, I was anxious about even more surgery for Barry. This was to be operation # 5, only six months on the heels of the last one, and the third one in less than a year. How many more operations could he—or I—take?

As we made our way off the potholed Detroit freeways and back onto Beaubien, we could see our familiar high-rise looming off in the distance. My stomach churned the minute it came into view. But this time the weather was sunny, the grass —what brief remnants of it we could see amidst the abandoned buildings —was green, and the leaves on the trees gave the place a different cast. Unlike in December, it no longer looked like death warmed over. Now it was spring, and nature had come back to life. Maybe it wouldn't be so bad here after all.

Again, both our mothers flew thousands of miles to join us in Detroit for this next phase of our medical odyssey. As we all settled into our respective rooms at International Center/Guest Housing, we braced ourselves for what we thought would be a repeat performance of last winter.

But before his operation, Barry needed to undergo a slew of tests. First was an endoscopy. Another spate of tests followed. One knocked him out, another bloodied him up, and a third required him to keep his right leg motionless and elevated for a grueling six hours. The nurses seemed confused about what to do with him. He was an outpatient, but he was jerked around from one hospital room to another until he landed in the right spot, where he was parked for the rest of the day.

"How tall are you? How much do you weigh? When is your birth date?"

He must have been asked these questions at least 20 times that day, and by at least 20 different people. I don't think he grew any taller, weighed any more, or turned any older during the several hours that he was there. And in this high-tech era, neither of us could figure out why this information was not computerized. It seemed like the height of inefficiency.

In the meantime, Dr. Fromm was flying in from South Africa, where he had given a series of lectures. He had explained this to us earlier over the phone, so it was no surprise. No doubt he would be back in Detroit in time for Barry's operation, and he promised to give us a call at International Center the night before the surgery. Surgery was scheduled for 7:30 a.m. on June 6, D-Day. About 10:00 the evening of the 5th, our telephone rang. I picked it up. It was Dr. Fromm, who had now returned from his travels.

"Welcome back, Dr. Fromm!" I said. "We'll look forward to seeing you tomorrow. We're so glad you're willing to do this operation for Barry."

"I'd like to talk with him about that. You see, there may be a change," he said.

With that I turned him over to Barry. I felt my knees start to buckle, and my body began to ache.

"On the basis of the test results presented to me, I can see complications," the doctor explained. "But I need more time to go over everything carefully later this evening, and then make a decision about how to proceed. I still hope to operate in the morning. But you should know that there's a chance that I may not be able to do the operation. Let's all meet in my office at 6:00 a.m. By then we'll know exactly what to do."

When he hung up the phone, Barry felt perplexed but managed to sleep reasonably well. Not me, though. By now my stomach was really churning. No operation at all? Neither of us had remotely conceived of this possibility. It couldn't be true! My head was spinning, and I tossed and turned all night long. I must have eked out a few hours sleep, but they were fitful at best. When dawn began to break, I was already awake. It was time to face the day ahead: D-Day.

We gathered our entourage and walked over to Harper Hospital. Even though it was only 5:45 a.m., the sun was up high enough so that we didn't need a security escort. We entered through the rear of the hospital and found our way to Dr. Fromm's office. After the past few days in this alienating medical maze, it was a pleasure to see his familiar face. All four of us had grown to admire Dr. Fromm.

He greeted us all warmly and asked us to have a seat. I took a brief look around his neatly appointed office, with its wooden bookcases and miniature sailboat. I could see some scans on the light tables behind him. And I could tell from the look on his face that something might be amiss. He asked us to take a look at the scans. As it turned out, he explained, the problem was not so much the amount of cancer in

Barry's liver, though the cancer had definitely grown since December. Rather, it was that too many of the tumors were located in precarious spots. And surgery would risk puncturing a number of crucial blood vessels.

"I simply can't do it," Dr. Fromm said. "It's not worth the risk. I wish we had known this earlier. But we needed to see the results of the tests first. And the tests needed to be done just before the operation, because otherwise the situation could change in the meantime. So I'm canceling the operation."

His words hit me like a ton of bricks. Although I sat there calmly, jotting down notes in my diary, my head was reeling.

"This can't be true!" I said to myself. "This must all be a bad dream!"

And how did Barry react?

> At this point I began to wonder whether this trip to Detroit was even worth it. After all, a year and a half earlier, Dr. Curley had reached the same conclusion, that the liver was inoperable. Of course, Dr. Curley didn't think the greater omentum and belly cavity could be operated on successfully either, while Dr. Fromm demonstrated that they could be. So, at this point, I was a little confused and beginning to feel that the situation might indeed be hopeless.

However, Dr. Fromm made it clear that in lieu of surgery, he had one other possible alternative in mind for that day: a hepatic infusion. This involved injecting Barry's liver with alcohol, a practice, we were told, that is often used in Japan. Dr. Fromm made it clear that the alcohol would be concentrated only on those parts of the liver that were malignant. In any case, it was worth a try. He told us to come back to the hospital later that morning. In the meantime, I felt a sudden urge to escape from the confines of the hospital.

As we made our way out the hospital maze, we heard a frantic, high-pitched voice at our heels. It was a nurse chasing us from the other end of the corridor.

"Mr. Riccio! Mr. Riccio! Where are you going?" she shouted. "You're supposed to be in surgery today!"

She raced down the hallway, finally catching up with us.

"But Dr. Fromm just canceled the operation," Barry told her.

"I don't see that in my records," she explained, catching her breath. "They say that you're still on for this morning. And the operation is to begin at 7:30. We're all waiting for you in the operating room! Hurry up! You'll be late."

"But we just came from the doctor's office," Barry said. "He just told us so. It's definitely off."

She must have thought that Barry chickened out. With a puzzled look on her face, the nurse made a U-turn and sped off. The sounds of her footsteps echoed down the long corridor. Watching her silhouette against the eerie fluorescent lights, the four of us could barely contain ourselves. We each started laughing uncontrollably.

But as we walked out the hospital doors once again my head was spinning. By now it was only about 7:00 a.m., and I had been up for just two hours. My lack of sleep the night before already began to take its toll. And the drastic turn of events suddenly began to hit me. My body ached from head to toe. I felt as if a hammer were pounding on both sides of my head. That sensation remained with me all day long.

When we returned an hour or so later, we followed Barry all over the hospital. Even though his status was now switched from inpatient to outpatient, he still had to be readmitted and was forced to fill out even more paperwork.

Later we met another attractive blonde doctor who worked with Dr. Fromm and seemed to know exactly what was going on. This was reassuring.

"The hepatic infusion will take at least two hours," he said. "Why don't the rest of you go upstairs and get something to eat? You can come back and meet us when it's all over. And let's see if it works. If it does, Barry could come in regularly to be injected over a period of several weeks."

"Weeks?" I thought to myself. "You've got to be kidding! How much longer would we be here? One minute we find out that the operation is called off altogether. That means our stay in Detroit will be cut short. But the next minute we find out that we may need to be here for weeks. What kind of a roller coaster ride is this?"

So we said good-bye to Barry, who was waiting patiently on the gurney. By now we were hungry for lunch, so we headed on up to Wendy's for a bite.

By the time we returned to Radiology, we found Barry sitting up in his gurney, waiting for us. I could tell instantly from the look in his eyes that now something else had gone wrong.

"Where have you been?" he said. "I've been waiting for a long time."

"We were told to come back in two hours. So here we are," I said. "What happened?"

"It didn't work," Barry said. "This time there were even more tests, and I even got to see my liver on a computer screen. But the doctor came to the conclusion that the hepatic infusion could not take place. The reason for this was that I had a rather large tumor growing out of my portal vein. Apparently that vessel transports nearly 80% of the blood to the liver. So we're back where we started."

By the end of the day, we ended up back in the hospital room, waiting to meet with Dr. Fromm. He walked in around 5:00. Barry asked him if there were any other options left. He thought of one remote possibility, but the next morning even that was no longer a live option.

Barry then asked Dr. Fromm the inevitable question, "Just how much time do I have left?"

The doctor hesitated to respond, perhaps because our two mothers were in the room, not to mention me.

"No one knows," he said. "But definitely do keep in touch. I want to follow your progress. You've all had a very long day. Now I just have one piece of advice: go out and enjoy a nice dinner. And have a safe trip home."

We each shook his hand warmly and said good-bye. And what was Barry's reaction?

> At one level, I was overwhelmed by the news. I was
> enervated. At the same time, I was no more nervous than I had
> been earlier. To some extent, I even felt relieved, in as much as
> the suspense was now over. At least I would not have to
> undergo another operation, and could live —if only for a year
> or so —a fairly normal life. At the same time I was eager to get

out of the hospital. And since I had not had a good meal for several days, I was actually rather hungry.

So we followed the doctor's orders. Within an hour I was behind the wheel in rush hour traffic heading out to Dearborn. There we tracked down a popular Lebanese restaurant that our neighbors, Carole and Tino, had recommended. By the time we got there it was mobbed. A line of people overflowed out the door and onto the sidewalk. When our turn came, we squeezed our way through the crowd and into a booth. The steady beat of drums and high-pitched sounds of clarinets blared in the background. Colorful posters of Beirut lined the walls. Toddlers, teenagers, parents, and grandparents were all wolfing down their dinners. Little did any of them know where we had just come from, or what we had been through. But that was o.k. Somehow seeing people going about their everyday business was reassuring. It was a relief to get back to planet earth. Although I was exhausted, my shish kebab, pita bread, and Diet Coke gave me a second wind.

As Barry put it, "it was a very enjoyable meal, and it seemed like a very normal event in spite of the very abnormal circumstances behind it."

It was the best medicine the doctor could have ordered.

Theoretically we could have packed our bags and returned home to Illinois the next morning. But a more practical issue caused us to stay in Detroit for a few more days: Felicia's airplane ticket. By leaving early, she would have incurred a penalty that she was unwilling to pay.

So we became tourists. We rode out once again to Dearborn, this time to Greenfield Village. There we saw the Henry Ford Village, a popular attraction with replicas of famous events from American history. Even though the village idealized Henry Ford, Barry despised him, reminding us that he had been a virulent anti-Semite and a racist, among other things. Yet for the rest of us, compared to Harper Hospital, the peaceful slice of Americana portrayed by Greenfield Village was a soothing remedy.

Another day we crossed the border to Ontario, Canada, and discovered the city of Windsor. We drove all over the city, impressed with its scenic waterfront parks, its traditional British gardens, and its pedestrian-oriented main street. There we spotted out a tiny Thai restaurant tucked away in a basement. The food, especially my coconut soup, was scrumptious. Ever since I had first tasted it, I loved Thai food. It instantly became my favorite ethnic cuisine. Its artistic presentations and mellow flavors always put me in a good mood. And since Thai restaurants had not yet hit Champaign-Urbana, whenever we were in Chicago or any other large city, I always sought them out.

One of Windsor's major attractions is its huge casino. None of us had ever been fond of gambling. Yet as the day wore on and we strolled along the waterfront, with its old-fashioned Mississippi Riverboat casino perched prominently at the dock, Mom and I had second thoughts. Temptation drew us in. While I lost my money in record time, Mom's machine started gushing out coins like a waterfall. She put some of them back in, and even more poured out. I could see her eyes light up and her face beaming each time she pulled the lever. It was her lucky day. We both began laughing and couldn't stop. And by the time we left, she had won over $40, half of which she gave to me.

After visits to Birmingham and Cranbrook, sites familiar to us from our previous stay, we said our final good-byes to International Center/ Guest Housing and took Felicia to the airport. Barry, Mom, and I began our trip home, making a detour to Holland and Saugatuck on the west coast of Michigan. Mom had never seen that area before, and I was looking forward to showing her some of our favorite vacation haunts. On our way south through Indiana we made another detour to a favorite Thai restaurant of ours off the freeway. After yet another coconut soup, I was in heaven. Later that afternoon, after our final stretch on the desolate prairie of I-57, we finally made it back home. When I walked into our living room, it felt as if an old friend were waiting to greet me.

Yet even now the memory of June 6, 1996 remains firmly etched in my mind. As I lay in bed that night, snippets of the day's events rolled through my head, like scenes from a Kafakaesque nightmare. That day would go down in history as one of the worst days of my life.

It was yet another body blow —perhaps the heaviest load we had to bear so far. The sudden turn of events left us all devastated. I felt so sorry for Barry, and could only imagine how disappointed he must have been. Yet I also pitied both our mothers, who had flown thousands of miles and spent hundreds of dollars for an operation that was never to be. And I felt badly for Dr. Fromm. He had genuinely tried to help us, but now was rendered helpless himself. Ever since we had first met him back in December, the four of us were among his biggest fans. And we still felt the same way about Dr. Curley, too. Both were so dedicated, so competent, so professional —truly tops in their fields. And they were so approachable, so humane, so patient, and so considerate. We couldn't have asked for better doctors. But now even our second lifeboat appeared to be sinking.

As our eyes wandered over the dreary Detroit skyline, we knew that once again, we had reached another impasse. That machine gun was aiming right at us. The bullets continued to fly. But could we still keep dodging them? Sooner or later we were bound to be hit.

Yet early the next morning Barry made a phone call to California that would change our lives. A while ago, Dad had sent us an article from *The San Diego Union-Tribune* describing some promising studies at Scripps Research Institute in La Jolla. Barry would read a similar piece later in *The New York Times*. Scientists at Scripps, led by a Dr. David Cheresh, were pioneering a brand new treatment for cancer: an antiangiogenic approach which attempted to cut off tumors from their blood supply. It would inhibit the birth of new blood vessels, thus cutting off nourishment to the cancer cells. But it was probably too early to be tested in humans.

In fact, I had called the staff at Scripps back in October 1995, just as we had returned from MD Anderson, having reached our first medical cul-de-sac. At that time, I reached Dr. Cheresh's assistant.

She explained, "The new drug is known as LM-609, and it is still in the laboratory, preclinical stages. We're not yet certain when it will be ready for human trials. No protocol has been established. A small biotechnology firm in Sorrento Valley, called Ixsys, has licensed it to make synthetic antibodies. Why don't you call back in about six months or so when we'll know more?"

And now it was already June. Here is Barry's version of events.

> When I woke up that morning, even though I was still
> mentally exhausted, I felt I owed it to myself to make that

phone call. A part of me did not want to make the call because I was wiped out. Yet another part of me couldn't forgive myself if I didn't dial that number. It was one thing to avoid having an operation. It was quite another merely to wallow in the status quo, especially when that status quo was still unacceptable to me. Finding out about antiangiogenesis therapy was hardly whistling in the dark. After all, I would not be dealing with some medical charlatan or panacea peddlers with half-baked ideas. Once again, I did not want to leave any legitimate stone unturned.

This was our last resort. By now, even I began to have my doubts about whether or not our quest for treatment should go on. But the next phase of our medical odyssey was about to begin.

CHAPTER FOUR

Go West, Young Man
(1996-1997)

"THE MEASURE OF A MAN IS THE WAY HE BEARS UP UNDER MISFORTUNE."
— PLUTARCH

On February 12, 1997 Barry made a dramatic departure from his home, his job, his wife, and his life in Illinois. He drove cross-country out to California to participate in the Vitaxin (also known as LM-609) clinical trial. My feelings about his leaving were mixed. On the one hand, if there were still any faint glimmer of hope, I wanted him to have it. On the other, if the trial proved to be a failure, that meant that we simply had fewer months left together.

After his initial call to the research team at Scripps in spring 1996, Barry was told to keep phoning until more information was available. He did just that. Eventually they put him in touch with the biotechnology company that would be sponsoring the study. Several calls later, he was told to contact the health care provider that would be administering the treatment. At that point, he established a relationship with Joy Hamer, the clinical oncology research coordinator at the Sidney Kimmel Cancer Center. She said he sounded like a good risk for the protocol, and that he should keep in touch regularly.

Even though we were still reeling from our disaster in Detroit, in July we managed to travel out to California. At first I doubted whether or not either of us could muster up enough energy for yet another journey, but in retrospect it was a wise decision. When some of our Bay Area friends learned that we were wavering about the trip, they made our airline reservations for us, paid for our tickets, and planned several events on our behalf. Never before had any friend of ours made us such a generous offer. Usually our trips to the Bay Area took weeks of advance planning, but this time I was so drained that I could barely pick up the phone. Acting as our travel agents, they gave us one of the best presents they could. Several were waiting for us at the San Francisco Airport. Some took us on a scenic hike at a nearby redwood forest, and others planned group get-togethers over dinner.

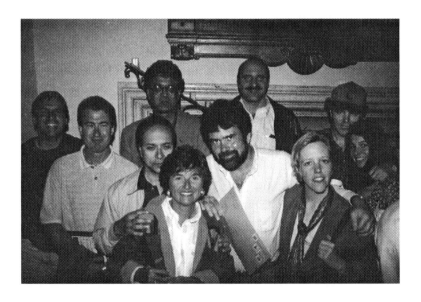

Friends planned a party at International House to celebrate our return to the Bay Area. They paid for our airline tickets from the Midwest. L–R back row: Dean Kardassakis, Peter Pinsky, Christopher Flores, Paul Speigel, Eric Cammarena, Christine Self. Middle row: Sankar De, Barry, Kate Harrison. Front row: myself. Berkeley, California; July 1996. (credit: Robert Englund)

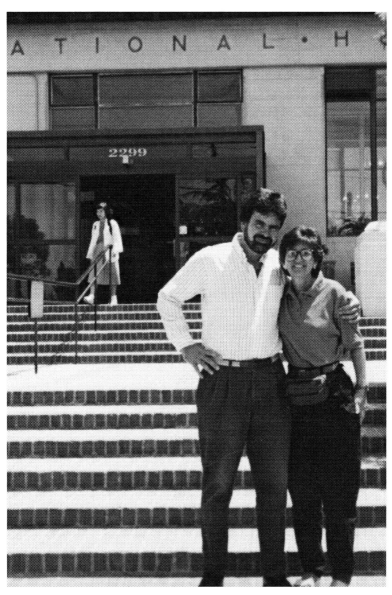

An earlier shot at the International House, University of California, where Barry and I had met as graduate students. Berkeley, California; July 1994. (credit: unknown)

Mid-week, our friend Eric had arranged a dinner for us at International House in Berkeley, where Barry and I had first met 20 years earlier. A slew of friends— many of them former I House residents themselves— were waiting for us on the front steps. After posing for photos, we made our way into the Dining Room for our meal, just as we used to do as students. We all sat outside in the courtyard where Barry and I had held our Northern California wedding reception. The I House staff offered us several bottles of wine to celebrate the occasion.

"Let's all have a toast to our good friends, Barry and Kathy," Eric said. "To their good health!"

As he raised his glass and continued with his short speech, I was moved to tears. Seeing so many of our friends gathered together in such a familiar place seemed almost magical to me. Others had done the behind-the-scenes legwork and all we had to do was appear. It was too good to be true. And as my eyes gazed around the courtyard I reminded myself that although we were unlucky in many ways, we were indeed fortunate to have such wonderful friends.

Later that evening after dinner, several of us toured the building. We suddenly got the urge to visit our old rooms and meet the current occupants. As we knocked on the doors of Room 700, Room 762, Room 644, and Room 494 (rooms that Barry and I had each lived in), we paused while the leery students slowly creaked open their doors.

"I used to live in this room back in 1976. We're a group of friends here for a mini-I House reunion. Do you mind if we come in and take a look?" I said.

The student peered into the hallway at our group, and replied, "Sure, go ahead."

Barry and I didn't think we would have been as trusting 20 years ago. We repeated this scenario at almost 10 different rooms, chatting with the new residents, learning about where they came from, what they were studying, and how they liked Berkeley. It was the frosting on the cake.

A few days later, our friend Barbara drove down from Oregon to join us in Berkeley. We always enjoyed staying at Eric and Robert's home perched high atop a hill overlooking the San Francisco Bay. It was a large, red brick Georgian mansion designed by the architect, Julia

Morgan, who also planned the famed Hearst Castle. Their home felt like Hearst Castle to us. That Sunday, our hosts took us out for a sailboat ride on San Francisco Bay.

Later that evening was the grand finale to our week in the Bay Area. Eric and Robert had planned a potluck and barbecue dinner for us in their backyard, a substitute for our annual picnic at the Palace of Fine Arts. Some 50 friends joined us. The atmosphere was festive. Eric had invited an opera singer and a guitarist to entertain us, and they played beautifully together. As Barry and I sat together on the couch, listening to their lovely songs, once again my eyes panned around the room. I was overcome with emotion. All the events of the past week flashed before me. And I wondered whether or not this would be the last time Barry and I would be here together at One Eucalyptus. Would our Bay Area friends ever see him again? Would this be their final memory of the former "King of I House?" Who knew?

As Dr. Fromm had told us, "Nobody knows."

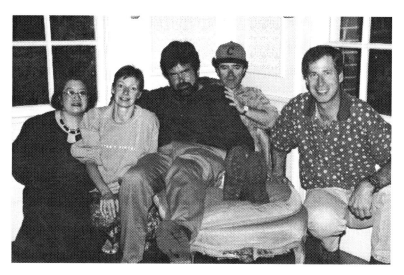

Robert Englund and Eric Cammarena hosted a party for over 60 Bay Area friends, the grand finale in a week–long series of festivities in our honor. They even hired an opera singer to entertain us. L–R: Monica Chan, Barbara Oberto, Barry, Eric Cammarena, Robert Englund. Berkeley, California; July 1996. (credit: author)

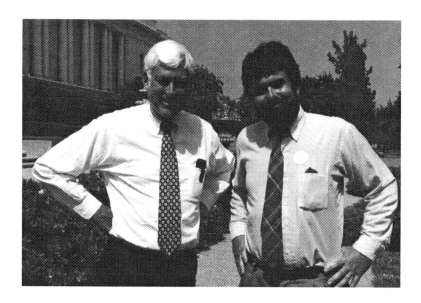

Fellow American intellectual historian Robert Scotheim, President of the Huntington Library, gave us a provate tour of his world reknowned research facilities and gardens. His favorable review appeared on the back cover of Barry';s book. He later wrote on behalf of Barry's tenure application. San Marino, California; July 1996. (credit: author)

We returned to Urbana in August. The next month Barry and I drove out to Topeka, Kansas for his Mid-America Conference on History. This was the conference that his two operations had caused him to miss twice before. Yet this time he was able to make it. Barry was thrilled to reconnect with his historian friends, and they were ecstatic to see him. On the way there, we celebrated my birthday in the historic section of Kansas City,listening to a local jazz group led by the brother of a good friend of ours. Compared to my melancholy mood the year before, this birthday was a huge improvement.

Fall semester was eerily normal, almost too normal in the wake of all that had happened earlier that year. Based on our past experience, we were now in the habit of bracing ourselves for bad news in the autumn. But this time, miraculously, no news was good news.

And in fact, this fall Barry had some even better news than usual— not medically, but professionally. On September 23, he received tenure. By then he had already been teaching in the Department of History at

Eastern Illinois University for five years, but he had only been officially on the tenure-track for a little over a year. Knowing of Barry's precarious health, and especially the medical impasse in Detroit only a few months ago, his colleagues bent the rules and accelerated the tenure review process— something virtually unheard of in academia. For Barry, tenure had been virtually a life-long goal. Here are his reflections about that time.

> I was very relieved and very happy because I had been dreaming of just this day for over 10 years, and thinking about it for nearly 20. It may not quite have been an obsession with me, but at times it veered perilously close to becoming one. In large measure, that was because of the fact that the job market in my discipline was so tight, and because there were not a few middle-aged men that I knew who had been in quest of a tenure-track position for a dozen or so years after they had been granted their Ph.D.'s.
>
> I felt lucky because I had finally made it. At the same time though, I felt badly for those that I knew never would. I still hope that my empathy for the proverbial gypsy scholar never fades. I was eager to celebrate with Kathy. When I came home, there were three congratulations cards awaiting me on the stairway, all of which were from her. Either she could not make up her mind as to which of the three she liked best or she may have thought that the trek towards tenure was three times as difficult for me as it should have been.
>
> The fact that I now had tenure, and perhaps just as importantly, the fact that my chair and so many others in my department pushed so hard for me to get tenure, canceled out a good deal of the emotional pain that I would have had during this period of time. For me, attaining tenure was almost as meaningful an objective as staving off death itself.

In October our friends Casey and Mary threw a party to celebrate Barry's tenure. I knew I should be planning the party at our own house, but before I could even get that far, they volunteered. And because I was still so wiped out, I was relieved. At the time, that was one of the best gifts anyone could have given us. About 50 friends arrived at the door, one by one, with gifts and cards for Barry. He was the man of the hour. The festivities spilled out onto the backyard deck, decorated with colorful candles and flowers. Our hosts had even hired a caricaturist who entertained everyone with his playful portraits. Once again I was struck at how fortunate we were to have such wonderful friends.

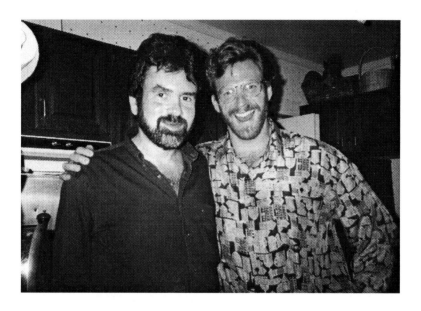

Barry with his former student, colleague, and friend, Casey Machula at a party to celebrate Barry's tenure at Eastern Illinois University. Champaign, Illinois; October 1996. (credit: author)

Right around this time, I signed a contract with the University of Illinois Press to complete my book manuscript, *Designing for Diversity: Gender, Race and Ethnicity in the Architectural Profession.* It was a body of research that I had been working on for the past few years, and it would continue to keep me occupied for even more. Writing came easily to me, and it was one of the most enjoyable aspects of my job. By now I had already written scores of articles as well as my first book, *Design Juries on Trial: The Renaissance of the Design Studio.*

All the while, however, I longed to write about issues outside my field as well. But with all my teaching, research, and administrative duties, I could never find the time. Plus on top of it all I was desperately trying to keep one step ahead of Barry's illness. The challenge of all else paled in comparison. Despite my having overcome the obstacles of promotion and tenure years ago, I felt uncomfortable with the narrow professional box into which I had been defined. Unfortunately academia seems to prefer it that way. We must all become experts, specialists in our chosen fields, and it is only through that work that we are rewarded. At major research universities such as my own, generalists are rarely valued. Yet the deeper we each dig into our box, the less we can see outside. Years later, even after I had leaped over another hurdle and become a full professor, I was still itching to pry open that lid, and jump out of that box.

And once again, Barry's birthday came and went. This time it was his 42nd. We celebrated at a local Indian restaurant with colleagues from his campus. Although it was a fun-filled evening, once again that same old question gnawed away at me: how many birthdays, if any, would Barry have left?

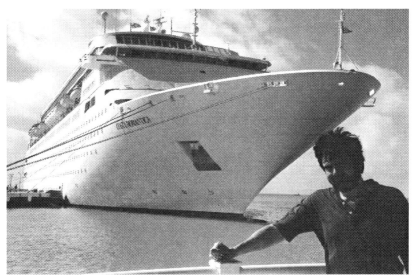

Barry at Key West, Florida. We didn't take a cruise but the ship made a scenic backdrop. November 1996. (credit: author)

Barry and I continued his birthday celebration over the Thanksgiving holiday in Florida. We took a short trip to Key West, a place neither of us had ever seen before. From our Bed and Breakfast, we bicycled all around the island. The trade winds were so strong that I had to get off my bike and walk a good distance, but I loved feeling that clean ocean air. We rode all around our neighborhood, marveling at the colorful Victorian architecture, and toured the lavish tropical estates of Ernest Hemingway and former President Harry Truman. Shortly afterwards, we drove up through the Florida Keys to Fort Lauderdale to visit my Aunt Helen.

We spent the Christmas season with our parents in Arizona and California. In light of our past two holiday seasons trapped in Houston and Detroit, we were grateful to be out of the medical scene, at least for a while.

While in San Diego we drove down to Chula Vista to meet with Dr. Jurgen Kogler. If Barry were accepted into the Vitaxin research protocol, Dr. Kogler would be his treatment doctor. We deposited medical records at his office and spent about an hour discussing Barry's case. Joy Hamer, the oncology nurse, informed us that the study was likely to begin sometime early that winter. Fifteen patients would be participating, and because Barry had called so early and so often, he was only number two on the list. During our meeting, I asked Joy two key questions.

"What was the best case scenario? And what was the worst case scenario?"

The worst case was obvious. If after six weeks of treatment and a test a few weeks later, Barry's cancer would continue to grow, he would be discontinued from the study and return home. By contrast, the best case scenario was that his cancer would remain stable, possibly even shrink somewhat, or ultimately— though this was highly unlikely— disappear.

"If any of these were the case, and I hope they will be," I asked, "Then what? Will he be continued in the study? What's to guarantee us that he won't be dropped like a hot potato?"

Joy reassured us that he would not be dropped. Little did I know at the time how critical my questions would be.

Even then, I could not fully comprehend all the different organizations that would eventually be involved with Barry's treatment. The drug, Vitaxin, was developed at Scripps Research Institute. Originally, it had been manufactured in Great Britain. Here in the US, Ixsys, a biotechnology company, was preparing it into a compound appropriate for humans. Sidney Kimmel Cancer Center was the organization administering the research protocol. The Food and Drug Administration (FDA) had to approve the protocol before it could begin. If the phase one clinical trial of Vitaxin proved to have no toxic effects, phase two could begin. The purpose of this next phase would be to determine the appropriate dosage of the drug. Phase three, administered to an even larger sample, could begin only if phase two had been completed successfully. The FDA would need to review the results of all three phases of the clinical trials before approving the drug for public consumption.

In addition to these four organizations, a fifth and sixth would be involved. The Vitaxin would be administered in the Sharp Infusion Therapy Center, and lab work and any follow-up complications would be taken care of at Sharp Hospital.

A few weeks later we were both back in Illinois, starting our spring semester. Barry told his department chair, Anita, that he might have to leave sometime in the middle of the term for California. At the time, he wasn't sure if and when he'd really be going, but he wanted her to be prepared just in case. It was impossible for me to even consider going out there with him. I was in the final term of my administrative job, and there was no way that I could leave. What was more, I had already missed enough days of work due to Barry's illness over the past few years, and didn't want to miss any more. But the thought of him driving cross-country alone worried me.

One of the highlights of the winter of 1997 was the production of Barry's play, *The Review*, the one he had written while recuperating from surgery over a year ago. At an outdoor back-to-school party in August 1996, Barry had mentioned it to Tanya, the wife of a retired history professor at Eastern. She runs the Charleston Alley Theater in a converted garage off the downtown square. Her creative touch transformed the tiny space into a New York-style loft apartment as the set for Barry's play. *The Review* ran for five shows at the end of January. It was coupled with another one-act play by Joyce Carol Oates, *Greensleeves*. Friends braved the icy roads from Champaign-Urbana and Chicago, and Felicia flew in from Arizona for opening night. Friends hosted a party for Barry after the play.

Once again we toasted, this time, "To Barry, the playwright!"

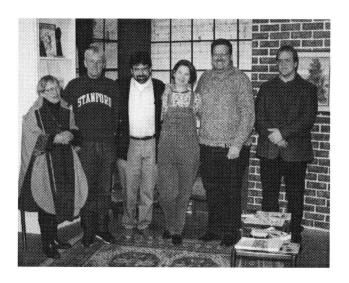

Barry with Tanya Wood, director, (L) and the cast of his play, The Review. The play was performed at the Charleston Alley Theatre just weeks before he drove out to California to participate in the Vitaxin clinical trial. Charleston, Illinois; February 1997. (credit: author)

On another snowy day Barry met with Dr. Michael Day, our family doctor. Barry sought an opinion about a small growth on his head which he had first noticed almost a year earlier. Dr. Day, like Dr. Johnson, thought the growth was probably a cyst but warned that given Barry's history, it could be cancerous. But both doctors suggested that he wait until he got out to California before pursuing the matter any further. When I first felt the protrusion, I couldn't help but think that it was yet another sign of the illness.

"This monster just wouldn't go away," I thought. "It's cropping up everywhere."

But how would I know? Soon afterwards, Barry phoned Dr. Curley to inquire about the results of his latest CT-scans. We had recently sent them out to him in Texas. I was worried about what he would say, as it had a bearing on when Barry should begin the Vitaxin protocol. If the scans looked o.k. Barry would teach through most of the spring semester and begin the study in April with a higher dosage of the drug. But if the scans showed any signs of trouble, he would need to start the treatment in February with the minimal dose possible.

As it turned out, according to Dr. Curley, "The latest CT-scan shows fairly substantial growth in a very short period of time— just between early December 1996 and late January 1997. If you wait to start the study in April, you might already begin experiencing pain and other symptoms. It's possible you might not even feel well enough to participate. If I were in your shoes, I'd go now."

Within days, Barry informed his chair that he would need to leave within the week. She looked concerned, but understood the situation, and wished him well. Soon we began to prepare for his departure.

He began to call his friends, one by one, to say good-bye. He bumped into others in the grocery store, in a restaurant, and at the post office. Whenever I heard snippets of these conversations, I felt a giant lump in the pit of my stomach, and I struggled to hold back the tears. I couldn't believe that in a few short days, he would be gone.

What bothered me most was the uncertainty of it all. What if after three months, nothing was accomplished? Then all this would have been a huge waste of time— precious time. Ever since Barry had fallen ill, I drastically cut my business travel schedule, passing up conferences and lecture opportunities that I would have jumped at in the past. What if something went wrong while I was away— another collapse in the bathtub, another emergency? Or what if I died in a plane crash? Could Barry face this deadly illness alone? Thoughts like that caused me to stay close to home. For years, spending quality time together had been my top priority.

Yet none of that seemed to matter now. It seemed that I was no longer essential. Barry was willing to undergo a separation. So should I. Once again, we faced another countdown. By now it began to feel as if my life were full of countdowns: the countdown to leave for Rochester in November 1993, the countdown for Houston in December 1994, the countdown for Detroit in December 1995 and again in June 1996. This next episode was just another ticking time bomb. Each night that drew closer to Barry's departure, I cried myself to sleep. Although we knew when he was leaving, we had no idea when he would return. The longer Barry succeeded in the protocol, the longer he would be away. The worse he did with the Vitaxin, the sooner he would be home. It was a Catch 22.

And for the first time, Barry had to stop working. Within weeks the official forms would arrive to certify that he was eligible for disability. Despite all that had transpired, when I saw those forms with Barry's name on them, it was heartbreaking. I couldn't help but think about the hundreds of job applications he had written and the piles of rejection letters he had received over so many years. There was no doubt in my mind that history was a cruel profession, and he deserved far better than that. Ironically, the job of his dreams—his tenured position— had finally been in his grasp, and now, because of a relentless illness, he had to let it go.

As the bags of travel supplies piled up in the hallway and I started packing up Barry's car, the finality of it all hit me. I felt like I was sending my husband off to war. My world was coming apart at the seams.

As I watched his car pulling out of our driveway for the last time, I braced myself on our front door, my face sticking to the glass. From the minute that I woke up that morning, no matter how hard I tried, I couldn't stop crying. A steady stream gave rise to a gushing river, then an overflowing flood of tears. I could barely watch as his car disappeared down Pennsylvania Avenue.

I couldn't help but wonder, "Would this new drug work? Or would all this be a waste of time? And would Barry ever return?"

For several minutes, I sat down on our living room couch, stared at the walls, and listened to the silence.

"That was it," I told myself. "The moment you have been dreading for so long is over. He's really gone! Now get a grip on yourself."

But I couldn't. I was devastated. Scenes from our medical odyssey flashed before me like a fast-forward film. Urbana, Rochester, Houston, Detroit. Now one more city would be added to this list.

Minutes later the phone rang. I could barely speak, but in the back of my mind I thought it might be Barry, so I picked it up. It was.

"Are you doing o.k?" he asked.

"Not really," I replied.

"Are you going into work today?" he asked.

"Not right now, that's for sure," I said. "If I feel up to it, I may go in sometime after noon. But at the moment, I need to stay right here. I can't go anywhere."

"I hope you feel better," he said. "Just think, I'll probably be back in a few months. And we'll see each other over spring break."

"Right. Drive safely. I'll talk to you later, after I check the weather forecast," I said as I hung up the phone.

I had promised to check the travel conditions, as a winter storm was brewing. Which way the blizzard was headed would determine which route he would take. It turned out that the snow was aiming right towards Arkansas, so at the last minute he changed his travel plans. But before Barry headed west, he went to Charleston. Even though it was only mid-February, it was his last day of school.

Just 10 minutes before his late afternoon seminar on Post-World War II America was to let out, the door opened. Surprise! Barry's history colleagues, a few philosophy professors, the Dean of Arts and Humanities, and several graduate students entered the classroom with their arms full of food and drink. His last class ended with a party. Anita and the others showered him with cards, cookies, candies, sandwiches, and even a few tapes for him to play during his cross-country trek. They had all secretly put together a farewell booklet on a "Go West, Young Man" theme.

It contained photographs of his friends at school, cartoons, travel tips, and parting words from each of them. In the centerpiece was a hand-drawn map by Rick Riccio (not related), Barry's colleague, who has exceptional artistic talents. The map showed a caricature of Barry driving across the USA, complete with his arrival surfing on the Pacific, wearing a Mickey Mouse cap on his head. After about an hour, they said their good-byes. Barry returned to his office, finished up a slew of memos, and tidied up his office. Finally, at 9:40 p.m., two colleagues helped him stash away his last-minute items into his car and watched him drive away.

Here are his thoughts at that time.

> As I drove away from the EIU campus, I thought of myself
> as being a star in some movie about a man going out West to

make it big. Only I was not going out to make money. I was going out to save my life. As I began driving towards St. Louis, I could not help but ruminate on the day, and especially on the evening event. In fact, I didn't think of California at all for at least an hour or so after leaving Charleston, so obsessed was I with what had just transpired. I then begin to think of where I should sleep that night, even though I was not the least bit tired.

About half an hour shy of St. Louis, I decided to stop at the Powhattan Motel in Pocahontas, Illinois. I had always called Kathy from there whenever I drove through that area on the way back from a conference or teaching out West. Unfortunately, for all the sentimentality, the motel is completely bereft of charm. At about 11 p.m., when I appeared at the front desk, I was nearly asphyxiated by cigarette smoke and deafened by the barks of a ferocious dog. After an interminably long minute or two of waiting a frumpy and bleary-eyed woman came to the desk. She checked me in and handed me my key.

The room was dark and ugly. I spent the next hour and a half reading and re-reading all the comments in the farewell booklet, and munching on a box of Frango mints that one of my colleagues had given me. I called Kathy to tell her that all was well. I also described the party at some length to her. She responded that she was glad she wasn't there, for she would have been unable to contain her tears.

The next morning Barry woke up late and continued on his marathon ride. When he reached the Arch at St. Louis, he called me from his car phone. We talked until he reached the west side of the city. He stopped to visit a good friend of his from Southwest Missouri State University, and further west in Oklahoma he stayed overnight at the home of another colleague.

Here is how Barry described his visit.

I was very tired, but I wanted desperately to hear how my friend was doing since his young wife walked out on him exactly a month before, after just over a year of marriage. That

night I slept like a baby and woke up in the morning to a
pleasant sight— sun. I had not seen any of it for several weeks.
Stan made me some English muffins and we had a pleasant
time discussing our future plans.

The next morning Barry took off for Texas. Around noon he
reached that infamous landmark, the Big Texan. Since it was lunchtime,
he ordered a 5-ounce steak.

"It wasn't as tasty as before and the beans were a little bland," Barry
said.

He decided to forego the 72-ounce steak, whose price had now shot
up to about $50. From the desert of New Mexico he phoned Joy to
give her a progress report on his whereabouts. He pulled over early that
evening so that he could travel through the majestic mountain scenery
by daylight. The next day he arrived in Phoenix where he visited his
family. On February 17, Felicia joined Barry for the last leg of his trip.
They ran into a heavy rainstorm in the mountains just east of San
Diego but arrived in time for Barry to check into Sharp Hospital at 5
p.m. for a blood drawing. His travels left him exhausted. The next day
he returned to Sharp to undergo several additional tests to prepare for
the protocol.

———•◆•———

Somehow I managed to drag myself into work the afternoon that
Barry left for California. Only one colleague at my research office knew
what had happened. When she asked me about it, I gave a curt reply
and quickly changed the subject. Even my research assistant who
worked with me on a daily basis, had no idea that Barry had gone. I
preferred to discuss it as a fait accomplis, once I had time to digest his
absence myself. One by one, my co-workers and friends learned of his
departure. I still couldn't bear to talk about it.

And whenever I walked into our empty house, reality set in.

"Get used to it," I told myself aloud. "You're living alone now."

Every time I drove my car and faced the empty passenger seat, I had
the same reaction. Although Barry and I talked at least once a day by
phone, I keenly sensed his absence. Whenever I opened a closet and saw
his crumpled clothes, or a shelf stuffed with his books, not to mention

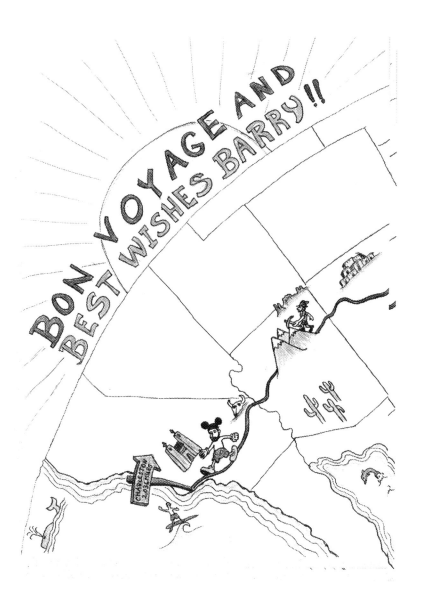

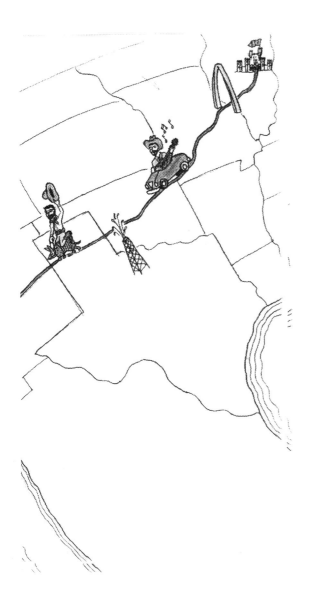

Barry's office partner, Rick Riccio, drew this caricature of Barry's upcoming cross-country drive from Illinois to California. It was part of a memory album that colleagues at Eastern Illinois University compiled for Barry's surprise going-away party. Charleston, Illinois; February 1997. (credit: Rick Riccio)

the many photographs of us scattered throughout our house, I was reminded of him. Although I maintained my teaching, research, and writing all with a semblance of normalcy, I knew deep down that life was far from normal.

After a few days I came up with an idea. Over the years we had filled several shoeboxes with post cards from our many travels to Maine and Michigan, to California and Colorado and Florida, and even to Hawaii and Greece. I began sending him a post card each day. Each one reminded us of the good times we had spent together. Soon they added to the decor of Barry's new room at Island Inn.

———•◦•———

On February 19, 1997, Barry began the Vitaxin study. He checked into the hospital for his first 90-minute infusion and spent the night there under observation by the medical team. In the meantime, I was back in Illinois, anxiously awaiting the news. Would Barry make it through the night? Would he be in a lot of pain? I recalled the list of possible side effects described in the research protocol. Blindness was one of them. So were loss of hearing, loss of mind, and death. Although that hardly made Barry blink, I found the list daunting. When I returned home that evening, I found a phone message on my answering machine. It was Barry.

> I'm calling from the hospital. I had my first dose of
> Vitaxin a few hours ago. So far it's going fine. My only
> symptoms seem to be a fever, a headache, some aches and pain,
> and a few chills. But after two Tylenols, I'm feeling much
> better. My mother was here earlier, and so were your parents.
> So was Joy Hamer, and so was the research doctor. Now they've
> all left. But don't worry about me. I'm doing alright.

That was the first week in what would be a series of countless medical appointments for Barry. Nurses drew his blood at 30 minutes, one hour, two hours, four hours, and eight hours after the initial infusion was over. Then again at 24 hours, 48 hours, and 72 hours. A week later he returned for his second infusion. This time he did not need to be hospitalized, but he still had to stick close to the clinic for the same schedule of blood drawings. It was a routine that would last six weeks. I wondered how other patients who were not in as good shape as Barry could endure that rigorous schedule of hospital visits. No sooner would he go home for a nap than it was time to drive back to the clinic again.

Felicia returned to Arizona in another week or two, but Barry was not alone for long. My parents lived only 15 minutes north, and they invited Barry over to the house a number of times. And soon after he left Urbana, I had contacted a small group of friends who lived in Southern California to inform them of Barry's new whereabouts and how to contact him. They all did. A steady stream of over 60 visitors traveled by plane, train, or car to spend time with Barry in San Diego. Because Barry was a stranger in a strange land, it was a treat to see familiar faces.

Although Barry's Vitaxin treatment seemed to have minimal side effects, he was still not spared of his illness and its defiant symptoms.

In early March, I began to realize that the "cyst" on my head was bothering me more and more. In fact, there were nights in which it was difficult to sleep. I discussed this with Joy Hamer and Dr. Kogler, and Joy reviewed the matter with a head surgeon at Sharp Clinic. The surgeon decided to do a little biopsy, as he put it, on my head. He seemed convinced it was a cyst and not a tumor, but he said that there was only one way to find out. So one afternoon Dr. Y anesthetized a small portion of my head and then began to scrape off my bump. I felt no pain because of the anesthesia but after a few minutes I sensed that some liquid was dripping down my neck.

"Am I bleeding at all?" I asked the doctor.

"Yep. You're bleeding like a pig!" he replied.

This did not reassure me, especially since roughly one-third of my brand new burgundy shirt would be saturated in blood within less than five minutes.

"That cyst was clearly a cancerous tumor," the doctor explained. "I'll have one of our girls clean you up." And then he disappeared

A gentle, sweet-tempered Mexican nurse spent a half-hour

washing both my shirt and head in peroxide and then wrap-
ping me up in bandages. When I emerged from the doctor's
office, a number of nurses in the clinic expressed shock.

"You look as if you stepped out of the pages of Stephen
Crane's *The Red Badge of Courage*." one of them said.

When I woke up the next morning, my sheets and
pillowcases were bathed in blood. It was quite a shock. The
pain was even greater now than it had been the previous night.
So I phoned Dr. Y's office and made an appointment. When I
met the doctor I told him that I needed some painkillers. It was
amazing to me that he had never prescribed them in the first
place.

That weekend our friend Peter flew down from Palo Alto. When he
first saw Barry at the airport, he was taken aback. Luckily he was able to
change Barry's dressing from time to time, a messy task that Barry could
not do alone. In between medical episodes, they strolled through the
Gaslamp Quarter, ate at a stylish Italian restaurant, and listened to jazz
at the Horton Grand, a stately Victorian hotel diagonally across from
Island Inn. It would soon become one of Barry's hangouts. Later that
weekend as the clouds loomed along the coast, they found sunshine in
Anza Borrego desert a few hours away. When Peter left that Sunday
night, he worried about leaving Barry alone. But Barry reassured him
that I would be out there in just a few days.

By the time I arrived for my spring break, Barry was feeling better.
His head was still bandaged. Although he had warned me in advance,
seeing him that way for the first time was a shock. When I had last said
good-bye to him in Urbana, it felt as if he were going off to war. Now
he even had battle scars to prove it.

I still must have looked pretty bad for one of the homeless
men across the street expressed some pity when he saw me.

"How'd you get to look that way? Did somebody hit you
in the head?" he asked.

I decided to make it easy on myself and merely nodded in
agreement. That made him feel even more sorry for me.

I had to wear a series of bandages for approximately three

weeks, and while it was awkward at times, I got used to it eventually. Though I was self-conscious in the beginning, over time I managed not to worry all that much about how I actually looked to others. Once again, I felt as if I were playing out a role in a movie script.

At first, I, too, was keenly aware of Barry's appearance. Wherever we went, I could see passersby do a double take. A few of the more curious types stopped to ask us what had happened. The minute we mentioned the word "cancer," they stopped dead in their tracks, speechless.

After a few seconds, one of them would say, "Oh, I'm sorry," and quickly walk away.

Yet none of this fazed Barry. If I were in this condition, I probably would have wanted to hide inside, but Barry wanted to be out and about as much as possible. So we went about our normal business.

I first saw Barry's apartment at Island Inn just as spring arrived on March 21, 1997. Little did I know then that within months, this tiny space soon would become home for both of us. I arrived in San Diego shortly after midnight. When I walked in the door to #380 I was pleasantly surprised.

When Barry completed his housing application for Island Inn back in January, I had added a handwritten note: "Cancer patient. Needs a unit with lots of sun, good view. May need to be in his room for extended periods of time. Thanks a lot."

Much to my amazement, the staff complied. Without a doubt, compared to almost all the other 200 units in the building, Barry's was one of the brightest.

Floor to ceiling glass lined the corner walls to the south and west. By day, sun streamed into the room, turning it into a greenhouse. We faced an ivory six-story condominium complex with lofts, bay windows, and street-level gardens. To the west were the twin towers of the Marriott Hotel as well as the Hyatt Regency. And from a small break in the skyline once in a while we could see the tall masts of navy ships cruising in the bay. A block away were the treetops from the Children's Park, an oasis of green mounds, cypress trees, and turquoise waters.

During my spring break, Monica flew down from San Francisco for a few days. She and I had known each other for over 20 years from Ida Sproul Hall, our college dorm at Berkeley. Throughout Barry's illness, she had been exceptionally kind to us. During our stay in Arizona for Christmas after Barry's MD Anderson operation, one of the first pieces of mail we received was a package from Monica. She had hand-painted a colorful banner with get-well wishes for both of us, complete with a sketch of the Golden Gate Bridge. That banner hung up in our bedroom ever since, and we thought of her every day. I later learned that just days before she mailed it she had been mugged in her parking garage and had her wallet stolen. I couldn't believe she could take the time to do something special for us under those circumstances. On another occasion she sent us a gourmet chocolate bar and one of her favorite recipes for chocolate cake. Right before Barry's last Christmas in Illinois, she had flown out to visit us in Urbana and she stayed for about a week. It was great to visit with her again in San Diego. We took her to see the flower fields in Carlsbad, a stunning display of ranunculus in stripes of red, white, yellow, gold, pink, and orange.

Soon after Monica left San Diego, Barry had another doctor's appointment. The surgeon told us that he could operate on Barry's head next week. Either that or he could wait until later. His excisional biopsy had only removed about 40% of the tumor, and the rest of it had to go. Although I was planning to return home at the end of the week when my spring break was officially over, I decided to extend my stay in order to be with Barry during his operation.

On April 3 he checked into Sharp Hospital once again. He would only be there for one night, which sounded like a piece of cake compared to all his other operations. Despite the fact that the surgeon had called the operation "no big deal," he was wrong.

My parents joined me while Barry was under the knife. We waited for several hours expecting to meet with the doctor. But he never showed up. He must have forgotten about us, but we never forgot about him. Finally, we learned from the receptionist that the operation was over and that Barry was already back up at 8 North, the Oncology Unit. So we raced up the elevator to find him.

By now I had already learned that any patient right after an operation looks like death warmed over. So I braced myself for the worst. But even my best efforts failed to prepare me for this. As we tiptoed into the

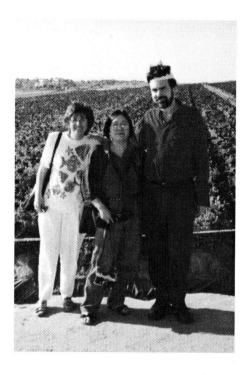

The two of us with Monica Chan at the Flower Fields. Barry's head tumor was bandaged for several weeks while he awaited surgery. Carlsbad, California; March 1997. (credit: unknown)

room I saw a body lying on a bed. But all that I could see of the face was a pair of eyes. Nothing more. His entire head, hair, beard, and even mouth had been wrapped in a gauze helmet, like a mummy. He looked just like the protagonist in the film, *The English Patient.* As I bent over to give him a kiss, I felt my knees begin to buckle and the blood gush right out of me. I was only seconds away from fainting. I darted over to the chair and lowered my head between my knees to get the circulation flowing. I tried my best to pull myself together. I didn't want to fall apart in front of Barry and my parents.

Here is how Barry described the aftermath of the surgery.

> It wasn't just that I had a huge bandage around my entire head and a good chunk of my face. It was also that I could barely speak because the bandage was wrapped around my chin so tightly.
>
> There was more. Whenever I got up to go to the bathroom, my leg began to bleed profusely. The surgeon had done a

skin graft there so as to replace the tiny hole in my head that
had been created as a result of my operation.

Once we returned to Island Inn, I instantly became his nurse, maid,
chauffeur, and secretary—roles that I would continue to play for many
months to come. The night before, from my parents' house, I was e-
mailing news of his fifth operation to friends around the country.
Within hours, an outpouring of get well wishes arrived on our computer.

A day or two after the surgery, Barry was not feeling any better. At
times his pain was excruciating. Late one evening while he was convers-
ing with an Illinois friend on the phone, he began to feel blood trickling
down his neck. He was still strapped up in his gauze helmet, and I
added even more bandages to the pile, but when we woke up the next
morning, we could see blood seeping through to the pillowcases. The
next day while taking his Saturday morning calls, blood began to leak
from his leg, spilling all over the carpet.

At this point I called an old college chum who lived in San Diego,
Dan, a doctor. They had seen each other shortly after Barry arrived, but
Dan had never seen him in this shape. Within hours he came to our
rescue. For nearly an hour, he helped change Barry's dressing and tried
to stop the bleeding. He also attempted to remove the blood from our
carpet with hydrogen peroxide, a trick he had learned from his medical
training. I bought sandwiches from a nearby restaurant and we ate them
on our apartment floor. When things seemed somewhat under control,
the three of us drove to the Embarcadero and took a short walk along
the waterfront.

The next day after yet another doctor's appointment, I made a
detour at a local drug store to purchase what appeared to be a lifetime
supply of bandages. After what we had been through over the weekend,
I didn't want to be caught off guard.

At this point the blood, and the pain, and the mess were
beginning to get to me, and I felt slightly depressed. At least,
though, the tumor had been entirely removed. So I was told by
the surgeon, who seemed immensely proud of his handiwork.
In fact, he seemed more interested in the engineering and

aesthetic triumph he pulled off rather than the patient whose life he had ostensibly saved.

A few days later, Barry had a needle aspiration biopsy of his abdomen wall. This was in the area where he had first felt a tumor in the late summer of 1996. It was an aggressive biopsy even though it was done with needles rather than razor blades, and the tumor bled intermittently for some time.

In the meantime while still in San Diego, I attempted to teach my class in Illinois through remote control over the Internet. My students and I were all at our computers on Tuesday and Thursday between 4:00 and 5:30 p.m. Central time, 2:00 and 3:30 Pacific time. I asked them questions about their reading assignment and waited as their comments came in, one by one. Then I responded.

During that time, a colleague of mine had sent an e-mail message asking if I could make my office available to the Secret Service. Vice President Al Gore was speaking in our School of Architecture gallery, and his staff needed a spot to set up. I was pleased to oblige, but asked if in exchange, they could leave me a souvenir of their visit.

When I returned to my office a few days later I found a photo of the VP, complete with a note, "Thanks for the use of your office. Al Gore." His picture has become part of my office décor ever since.

Later that week Felicia flew into San Diego. She was a welcome sight. There was no way I could stay any longer, and Barry needed to have someone close by. Although Barry was still heavily bandaged on the evening that she arrived, the three of us took off for a Taste of the Gaslamp. Twenty restaurants nearby offered small portions of their best items for diners to try. Barry's war-torn look attracted the crowd's attention, but it didn't faze him. Once they got a glimpse of Barry, some of the servers gave us special treatment. We gradually made our way through Fifth Avenue, sampling tidbits from several different eateries. It was like Halloween in April, a trick-or-treat for adults, and a wonderful way to take our minds off medical matters.

That Saturday morning in the pre-dawn hours, I scurried about our apartment, stuffed my worldly goods in my suitcase, gorged down my breakfast, and kissed Barry good-bye. He was lying in bed, fast asleep. With his bandages still strapped around his head, he looked like a prisoner of war. A wave of guilt swept through me. How could I possibly leave him like this? But how could I keep my job if I didn't? I was in the midst of a tug of war, pulled in two different directions. That yanking sensation gnawed at me many times since.

As my plane sat on the runway and I watched the fishing boats splash along the bay, scenes of Barry's latest operation flashed through my head. As the plane rose into the sky, tears began streaming down my face. The stress of the past few weeks began to take its toll. By evening, I was back home in Urbana, back to our empty house.

That night, as I went through my stack of mail for the past three weeks, I came across a memo from a colleague notifying me that the faculty search committee that I had served on was recommending that I be dropped. I was dumbfounded. Weeks before, I had spent hours reviewing the files and portfolios of over 50 candidates. In order to finish this task before spring break, I had come into school on evenings and weekends. I had taken my computer with me to California and was accessible by e-mail and by phone. Yet on this matter, no one had contacted me. It struck me that I was the only woman on the committee. Would they have done this to a male colleague whose wife was sick? I held the memo in my hand, reread it several times, and exploded into tears. I confronted my colleague about it that Monday after a faculty meeting.

"I received your memo," I said. "And I feel as if I have been treated unfairly. Why didn't you or any of your committee members contact me? All you had to do was send me an e-mail. I was only gone for three weeks, one of which was spring break. And it was certainly not a vacation!"

I could barely finish my sentence. Suddenly teardrops began flowing, and I could no longer speak. I was embarrassed at losing control in front of my colleagues, and I headed out for my car. Days later, my director intervened and I was soon reinstated on the committee. I served out my term and was pleased to see a top-notch candidate hired. Yet the debacle reminded me of how emotionally vulnerable I had become. I could handle the day-to-day tasks at work provided nothing went wrong. But one more event like that and I might really go over the edge.

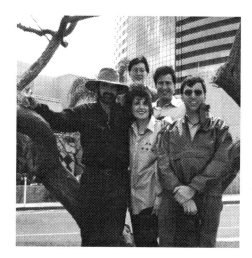

A steady stream of friends and relatives from across the country visited Barry in Southern California. Some came as many as ten times. His large Australian hat covered the scar from his recent scalp operation. L–R: Dan Chin, Joanne Lagos, Peter Pinsky, Dean Kardassakis. San Diego, California; April 1997. (credit: Aileen Smith)

While I was back in Urbana, several visitors came to see Barry in San Diego. On the weekend of April 19, Barry had a slew of company. Our friend, Joanne, arrived late Friday evening. Here is Barry's account of that weekend.

Joanne and I had a very pleasant stroll through the Gaslamp Quarter, and a leisurely chat at a little Italian eatery. She was struck by the European quality of the Gaslamp.

I said goodnight to Joanne close to midnight, but I was so excited to connect with a friend whom I hadn't seen for such a long time that I stayed up until 1:30 a.m., watching Alfred Hitchcock's *North by Northwest* for the fourth time.

The very next day around noon, Peter and his entourage descended upon 202 Island Avenue. With Peter were Aileen, a newfound significant other, Dean, our loyal doctor friend who had already visited me once before, and Daniel, yet another friend from I House days. I was utterly exhausted that day. After a hearty lunch at Cafe 222, we all went for a pleasant walk in the Seaport Village area. Joanne and I even did a little Greek dancing, although in all fairness, I should say that she did the dancing and I provided some comic relief.

In the early evening, all of us went to visit a friend of Joanne's in Coronado Cays, a part of the peninsula that I had never seen before. His house was beautiful. And more importantly, he made a massive salmon dinner for everyone, even though he had never met most of us before. Just before the dinner, we all went out on his little boat in San Diego Bay.

The next week my cousin, Sue, visited Barry. Later she and her husband, Jeff, would return with their four-year old son and new baby. Young Daniel was transfixed by the bright red cars of the San Diego Trolley, only a block away. After he returned home, he sent Barry a colorful drawing which we posted on the kitchen wall.

Soon afterwards, Colleen, another friend of ours from International House days, visited from San Francisco. She would make several more trips to visit Barry in the coming years. Colleen had been unusually kind to us throughout his illness. She often sent care packages full of treats such as healthy cookies and snacks, or fragrant soaps and hand lotions, items to cheer us up. She also sent us many cards and notes, not dwelling on the cancer, but rather just to let us know that she was thinking of us. Colleen had lost two of her brothers. One had been killed in the Vietnam War, and the other had died of AIDS. Years later she would lose her father to cancer. Perhaps because of her own experiences, she seemed to know just what to do to help others get through difficult times. And despite her personal tragedies, she always seemed upbeat. Over the years she had become my role model for dealing with adversity.

Unfortunately during this time Barry caught a bug.

Little did I know that I was beginning a two-week bout with bronchitis. Over the course of one week, I lost 10 pounds. I had a much diminished appetite when my friends Colleen Casey and Barbara Oberto came to see me in late April and early May. Barbara in particular took notice of how little I ate at my favorite Thai restaurant around the corner.

I did manage to go on an eight-mile walk with both of them. That probably exacerbated my condition. Because I did not have much energy, I did not go out much after Barbara left San Diego.

After his six infusions were over, on week #8, Barry had his first CT-scan out in California. Much to our surprise, the test showed that his tumors in the liver had stabilized, and the tumor in his abdominal wall had even begun to shrink. The wonder drug appeared to be working! Barry had called to tell me about it. I was ecstatic and started to cry.

"I can't believe it! I just can't believe it!" I said to myself. "This is too good to be true! Maybe that study did not turn out to be just a waste of time. If I knew back in February what I know now, I would have been delighted to see him drive off to California. 'Go, Barry!' I would have said."

I raced out the door to go for a walk. I needed to celebrate. I ran across Pennsylvania Avenue towards Carle Park. I felt as if a huge weight had been lifted from my shoulders. Suddenly as a cool breeze brushed against my face, everything in my path looked sharper and crisper than just hours ago. It was as if my contact lenses had been magically cleaned. Spring was in the air, and only now could I truly see it. Tulips stood taller, their reds, yellows, and whites somehow more vivid. Redbuds were beaming. Dogwoods were glistening. Even the sun was blazing brighter. The last time I had felt this way was almost two years before while swimming at the Rotary House pool, when we first learned that Barry's chemotherapy seemed to be working. It had been a long time since we had any good news. And I wasn't used to the sensation. I couldn't help but wonder: Could the past four years have been a nightmare, and would they soon be whisked away? Were we on the verge of a medical miracle?

Nonetheless, the good times could only last so long. In poet T. S. Eliot's words, "April is the cruelest month." And within only a few more days, it would be. That splendid day in April was but a blip on the radar screen. Barry explained why.

> On Friday, April 25, a little after 10:00 at night, I received a phone call from Dr. John Gutheil, who was in charge of the Vitaxin study. He told me that even though my tumors had stabilized, because I did not have a 25% or greater shrinkage, I could not be continued in the study. The biotechnology company was of the opinion that I should be dropped.

When I asked why the 25% or greater shrinkage was so important, Dr. Gutheil stated that that figure was spelled out in the protocol. I responded that I had never seen that protocol. I felt very bewildered and clearly somewhat bothered by this, though I did not take it as the final word.

This latest impediment spurred us into yet another desperate attempt to keep Barry alive. Luckily for us, that was the weekend our friend Colleen was visiting Barry. She just happened to be a lawyer and a judge.

I discussed the matter with Colleen the very next day. After she looked over my protocol and other papers the hospital had given me, she alerted me to the fact that in one of the documents, mention was made of Section 70707 of Title 22 of the California Legal Code. She suggested I look up the section in its entirety in the law library when I had a chance. When I did so a few days later, with the assistance of three librarians, I seized upon those provisions of the statute that bore most directly upon the matter of informed consent.

But I was not done. A few days later I consulted with another lawyer friend, Jan Bull, who carefully went over everything I showed him. He made the argument that I sacrificed a considerable amount of time, money, and psychological well being in order to risk my life by participating in this protocol.

Jan made the further point that Kathy had asked the $64,000 question of my nurse, Joy, when in December 1996, she inquired, "What's to assure us that if the drug is working, Barry would not be dropped like a hot potato?"

Joy assured us that if that were the case, Barry would not be dropped.

In addition, Jan was struck by the fact that the nurse's cover letter attached to the protocol stipulated that if my drug worked for me, I would be treated with continued doses of it.

"That," Jan said with the relish of a lawyer who had lived through the Watergate era, "is the smoking gun!"

What made the scene even more dramatic was that Jan was driving his car when he noticed this key passage.

Shortly thereafter, I wrote a draft of my letter to the biotechnology company that invented this drug. In doing so, I now had the encouragement of the Director of Clinical Oncology Research, John Gutheil, the same physician who had been the bearer of bad tidings on that night in late April. Now, once again, he was on my side.

Since I was up in the air about the future of my participation in the protocol, I became slightly depressed.

Saturday evening I attended a seder dinner at the home of a friend in Champaign to celebrate Passover. I had never been to a seder before, and I was entertained by all the rituals and songs. Later that evening Carole and I attended services for Greek Orthodox Easter. It was a moving ceremony, especially at midnight when all the lights in the church were extinguished and the priest arrived with a single candle, singing the chant, "Christos Anesti" ("Christ has Risen"). That Sunday afternoon, Carole and Tino had invited me home for a delicious Lebanese Orthodox Easter dinner. Their two sons, their daughter, and their spouses were all there for the occasion. I felt grateful not to be alone for Greek Easter and to spend this special holiday with friends. It had been a busy past few days, and the most ecumenical weekend of my life. But by Sunday night, I was exhausted. Then the telephone rang.

I first learned the news from my parents. They had phoned me that Sunday night to wish me a Happy Easter.

"Have you talked to Barry yet?" Dad asked.

"Not yet," I answered.

And so he told me. My parents seemed resigned to the company's decision.

"They must know what they are doing," Dad said. "You can't push them any further. They took him in the study from far away. They did their best for him. Most of these studies don't work anyway. They just use people like guinea pigs, just to test the drug."

"Yes, but what you're telling me doesn't make sense," I said. "First we find out that the drug is working so well that it's stabilized his cancer. But now they're tossing him out of the study. And they're sending him home to die.

"I'll tell you what this is. It's outrageous! It's unfair! I'm not letting this one pass!" I said as I hung up the phone.

The next minute I phoned Barry. We agreed to fight back right away, with every ounce of energy we had left.

On Monday I placed a phone call to our attorney in Champaign, and explained our situation at length. A few days later, Barry wrote a rough draft of his letter to the biotechnology company and faxed it to me at my office. I made some revisions and typed it up in my computer, and then faxed it over to our lawyer.

I wrote about our latest debacle to our two far-away doctors, Steven Curley in Texas and David Fromm in Michigan. Here is one of their replies.

5/2/97 e-mail from Steven Curley, MD, MD Anderson Cancer Center Houston, TX:

> Kathy,
> My only suggestion is that you communicate directly with the drug company and ask them to reconsider or allow treatment to continue on a compassionate IND [Investigational New Drug] basis. This is an unusual stance by the company.
> Steve Curley

I had never heard of the term, but it seemed to fit the bill. Later I learned that Barry had been informed of that option by a pharmacologist he met on the day he was first injected with the Vitaxin. We also turned to some other lawyer friends of ours— one in San Francisco, one in Orange County — and asked them each for advice. Calling attention to aspects of our plight that even we could not see, they each came to our rescue.

5/16/97 e-mail from Paul Spiegel, San Francisco, CA:

> ...Actually, to my mind, the issue is whether a company
> can induce a desperate patient into a toxicity study for an
> untried drug by promising continued treatment in the event
> that progress is shown, and then, after the fact, change the
> definition of progress to be able to drop him anyway. Alterna-
> tively, if they never changed the definition of progress, was the
> original definition made clear to Barry before he signed up? If
> he reasonably relied on their original promise that he would
> not be dropped, and if "progress" was never spelled out, [the
> biotechnology company] quite likely is contractually bound to
> provide further treatment if "progress" - however defined - was
> shown...

One of our friends had a sister in Washington, DC, who put us in
touch with an upper-echelon official at the Food and Drug Administration (FDA), the agency which oversees cancer protocols. The medical
staff in San Diego had told us repeatedly that the FDA was stringent
and did not look favorably upon any deviations from the standard
protocols. Barry contacted the woman at the FDA by phone and
described his dilemma.

"Go ahead and write your letter," she advised. "And see what the
biotechnology company says. I can see your point. And based on what
you told me, it certainly sounds as if you should be retreated. But if
they give you trouble, contact me again."

A few days later, she sent us some current news items and a direc-
tory of key personnel at the agency.

Relying upon all their suggestions, along with some input of my
own, Barry crafted a stirring letter pleading for his life. I finished typing
up the final version on my own computer in Illinois and faxed it off to
him in California.

"Good luck," I said to myself as I watched it disappear into the fax
machine. And there it went.

May 14, 1997

Mr. Z
Chief Executive Officer
Ixsys

Dear Mr. Z:

I am writing to request that you reconsider my case and
decide to retreat me as part of a continuation protocol for the
use of the drug, Vitaxin, which your company developed. As
you know, during the past few weeks, and after seeing positive
results from having treated me with Vitaxin during Phase I of
this clinical trial, my doctors at Sharp Health Care have
repeatedly recommended to you that I be continued in this
protocol. Apparently Dr. John Gutheil, Director of Clinical
Oncology Research, who is overseeing the protocol, has made
the case on my behalf to Ixsys at least three times to date. But
each time, your company has refused to continue my treatment....

As you know, I am a terminal cancer patient. I have
leiomyosarcoma, cancer of the stomach muscle lining, which
has spread to the liver and elsewhere. I was first diagnosed in
September 1993. Since that time, I have had five cancer
operations, six months of chemotherapy, and have been taking
numerous vitamins and herbs. I have been treated on numerous occasions for my illness at Carle Hospital in Urbana,
Illinois, where I live, met with doctors at the Mayo Clinic in
Rochester, Minnesota, and been treated several times at the
MD Anderson Cancer Center in Houston, Texas, as well as at
Harper Hospital in Detroit, Michigan. To the best of my
knowledge, I have outlived most cancer patients in similar
situations. As of May 7, I have completed Phase I treatment in
Sharp Health Care's antiangiogenesis/Vitaxin program in San
Diego. The procedure appears to have been largely successful,
at least from an educated lay person's point of view, inasmuch
as my tumors are no longer growing, and in some cases are
actually shrinking. At this point, this is the best news my

family and I could have hoped for. It would be even better news for all of us if I could be retreated as soon as possible, now that my participation in Phase I is behind me.

Prior to coming out here, my tumors had generally been growing at a rather moderate rate, although there had been "fairly substantial growth," in the words of one of my oncologists, between early December 1996 and late January 1997 alone. Considering that I was enrolled in a Phase I protocol, the primary purpose of which is to determine the toxicity of particular drugs, and that I received the minimally permissible amount of Vitaxin, I responded quite well indeed. Because of that response, I believe I am entitled to further injections of Vitaxin for the following reasons.

To begin, in order to participate in this clinical trial, I incurred significant expenses in driving out to San Diego and living here for at least a quarter of a year. Not only did I leave my spouse behind in Illinois; I also left my job as an Associate Professor of History at Eastern Illinois University, at least temporarily.

Last year, I had repeatedly contacted your company as well as the Sharp Clinic medical staff in the hopes of being admitted to the study. But I was also anxious to come because several of the medical staff informed me that, in the words of one of them, I "would not be dropped like a hot potato" if I showed signs of progress. Of course, progress is a relative matter. My reading of the latest advances in the cancer wars suggests that it is perhaps more realistic for patients to think of cancer as a chronic disease that can be contained, rather than as an illness that must either kill or be killed. I might add that the cover letter (dated 1/24/97) attached to my original protocol and consent form did stipulate, "The protocol for continuation of TX [Vitaxin] calls for an injection once every three weeks as long as it continues to work."

Which brings us to the all-important question, namely, what does it mean for a drug to work? I only learned a couple of weeks ago that 'work' meant remission, and remission by a certain amount. To be sure, the original protocol said something about remission being the ultimate aim, but it also stated that the immediate objective was to "inhibit the spread of the cancer." I was only informed in the tenth week of the program that the specific criteria for retreatment were spelled out in a continuation protocol. This document remains something of a mystery to me, for I have never laid eyes on it. Surely, I could not have been expected to know in advance of my trip out here that, as Dr. Gutheil told me, a good many medical protocols define a "minimal" to "partial response" as a 25-50% reduction in the cancer found throughout one's body, and mine was no exception. Had I known that, I might not have been as receptive to the idea of disrupting my career and family life as I was.

You are probably familiar with Title 22, Section 70707 of the California Administrative Code. It is, in essence, a bill of rights for patients. And it puts a particularly strong emphasis upon the patient's right to be fully informed as to the implications of all medical procedures. I now have to wonder if I really gave "informed consent" after all. Of no less significance, to my mind, Section 70707 also speaks of ensuring the patient "reasonable continuity of treatment."

At this point, you must be saying to yourself that "This patient's argument is with Sharp, not with us." I can certainly understand how you would arrive at such a conclusion. But it is my belief that Sharp Health Care/Sidney Kimmel Cancer Center is acting, in effect, as your agent. You are the sponsoring company, you are paying for the study, and your company's name appears at the very bottom of the original protocol's first page. Without you, the drug would not even be in existence. Moreover, every single one of the physicians associated with my case, as you well know, has recommended that I be retreated. They have been consistently supportive. My oncologist and surgeon at MD Anderson Cancer Center finds your position "unusual." Thus I have no quarrel at all with the medical community.

In the end, you will probably come back once more to the language of the protocol. I can only say that such protocols can be revised. More to the point, I can even be treated outside the protocol. This happens with cancer patients all the time, including many who are being seen at Sharp Clinic.

In closing, let me say that I appreciate all the work you have done in bringing into the world this very promising drug, Vitaxin. I would be even more appreciative if you would allow me to be retreated. I believe I am an excellent candidate who would advance your company's goals, and it is in your company's best interests, as well as mine, for Ixsys to continue to provide the treatment to me. You could learn a good deal from my case; moreover, other than the cancer, my general health is good. If Vitaxin proves to be truly effective for me and other people, we all stand to benefit, and you will be sitting on a gold mine. The longer it works, the better off we will all be. This is not yet the eleventh hour for me, but the bell is tolling.

I need to hear from you by Tuesday, May 20. Please respond in writing to my San Diego address: Island Inn, 202 Island Avenue #380, San Diego, CA 92101; fax: (619) 232-4183. If I do not hear from you by that date, I will presume that you will not be continuing me in the protocol, and at that point, I will have to look at all my other options. I eagerly await hearing from you.

Thank you.

Sincerely,

Barry D. Riccio, Ph.D.

Within a day or two of our deadline, we received a response by fax. It turned out that during the intervening period, the CEO to whom we had addressed the letter had been toppled. The new staff at the biotechnology company was moved by Barry's letter, and they were willing to reconsider. They agreed to pay for Barry's next CT-scan and base their decision on the results.

The May CT-scan showed that during the period while Barry had been off the Vitaxin— over about six weeks or so— his cancer had gotten worse. In fact, during this time the protrusions in his abdomen enlarged substantially, and the cancer in his liver had grown. Once again Dr. Gutheil made Barry's case, but this time with even more powerful ammunition: when Barry had been on the drug, he was doing well; but when he was off the drug, he was not. Weeks later, the same day that I returned to San Diego, Dr. Gutheil called Barry.

"I have some good news for you," the doctor said. "The company has agreed to retreat you. We're keeping you on the protocol on a Compassionate IND basis."

Barry recalled his feelings at that time.

> I felt relieved if not ecstatic that I won my victory. What I did not realize, though, is that it would take another four weeks before I could receive the drug again. Why? Because there was an inordinate amount of paperwork involved in writing up yet another protocol for me.

Finally, in late June, Barry began the Vitaxin protocol: round #2. The suspense was over. Our latest battle had been won. In our never-ending medical odyssey, it was a critical turning point. Once again, we had been forced to muster up our might. And once again, Barry's life was at stake.

The intense pressure of it all weighed on us like a ton of bricks. Our luck had changed, and success was finally in our grasp. But all too soon, another obstacle was thrown directly in our path. We hit another blockade. Our latest flurry of letters, faxes, e-mails, and phone calls had been enervating. After almost four years, what little strength we had left was slowly oozing out of us, trickling away, just like a tumor. Yet oddly, this most recent struggle had been energizing, too. Like players in a fencing match, we were forced constantly to be "on guard." When the sword struck, we had no choice but to rally and fight back.

Together, we had leapt over yet one more hurdle. The marathon runners had not yet run out of steam.

CHAPTER FIVE

Turmoil and Tranquility
(1997)

"A GEM CAN NOT BE POLISHED WITHOUT FRICTION,
NOR MAN PERFECTED WITHOUT TRIALS."
—CHINESE PROVERB

In late May 1997 I returned for another three-week stay in San Diego. Barry and I celebrated our 17th wedding anniversary at a jazz festival in the Gaslamp Quarter. The tunes of Dave Koz's saxophone and Jesse Cook's guitar filled the streets. The enthusiastic crowds spilled over our neighborhood. It was a festive day.

Given the nature of Barry's illness, I had often wondered whether or not we'd make it to our 14th wedding anniversary, or to any other, for that matter. Knowing that our days together were numbered, we began celebrating our anniversary on the 24th of every month. Why wait for an entire year to pass, when we might never get there? So reaching our 17th anniversary was a milestone. And knowing that Barry would now continue on the Vitaxin protocol, we had even more reason to paint the town.

Later that week we took a ride in San Diego Bay on Gondola de Venezia, a hand-built replica of an authentic Venician craft. Our friends Eric and Christine, who had driven down from Berkeley to see us, joined us on the boat. We started our ride a half-hour after sunset. Barry and Eric were joking with each other, just as they used to do in their rooms at International House over two decades ago. The stars were out, the sky was a deep blue, and the lights from the marina were twinkling. As our gondolier guided us through the narrow inlets of the bay, the four of us munched on antipasto, sipped a bottle of wine, and listened to Italian folk tunes. I could think of no better way to celebrate our anniversary.

Our street, Island Avenue, had its own romantic charm as well. Our favorite sounds were the clip-clop of horses from the Cinderella Carriage rides. Their route was right down our street. These white carriages, with their shiny wooden spokes and bright headlights, were landmarks of the Gaslamp Quarter. They looked as if they had leapt right out of a fairy tale. Drivers decked out in dark capes and top hats guided dark brown horses with white hoofs. Wide-eyed children, young couples, and even brides and grooms all curled up in their blankets, paraded outside our window. Whenever I heard them coming, I ran to the window to watch them go by.

From time to time we heard high-pitched bells from the pedicabs, a novel form of transportation that had recently caught on in the Gaslamp. From their oversized, bright red tricycles, drivers would ring their bells to entice potential passengers.

In the mornings we were awakened by the sounds of stacking tables and chairs onto the sidewalk at Cafe 222, a popular eatery adjacent to Island Inn. The clinking of glasses and silverware would also wake us up from time to time. But I never minded them, and for me, they were better than any alarm clock. The tiny cafe has only six tables inside and four outside. Every morning customers would line up along the entrance, reading newspapers and studying the menu. Weekends were by far the busiest. On Sundays crowds of conventioneers with look-alike nametags, athletes refueling after their early morning runs, and parents with toddlers in tow waited patiently for a table. All were drawn by the cafe's famous waffles, French toasts, and hash browns whose aromas wafted into our windows.

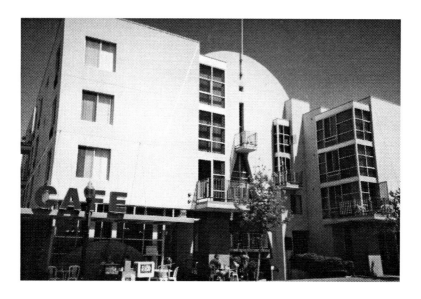

Island Inn became our home for over two years while Barry was receiving medical treatment at Sharp Hospital and Clinic. Our 300 square-foot studio was #380, second set of windows from the top on the right. San Diego, California; July 1997. (credit: author)

During those three weeks we discovered Art Tix, a booth which sold same-day half-price theater tickets, only a few blocks away. We frequented it often. From Island Inn, a good deal of the shows were only a short walk away. One of my favorite plays was *Boomers*, a musical about the Baby Boomer generation written by a local playwright. Another was "Buddy," featuring the rock and roll music of the 1950's with such classics as "Chantilly Lace," "Peggy Sue," and "La Bamba." As Barry had long been a theater buff, live entertainment became a diversion for both of us. The world of drama became yet another Great Escape.

That same month we attended Thiranixia, the opening of the doors of Saints Constantine and Helen Greek Orthodox Church in North San Diego County. This new church had been in the works for 19 years. Dad was the consulting architect, and Father Phillips, the priest who married us, still headed the parish. I felt so pleased for both of them and for all the parishioners who struggled to see their dreams come to fruition. The Bishop from San Francisco officiated, and hundreds joined in the ceremony.

But the three weeks whizzed by and soon it was time again for me to leave. I had a one-month summer appointment on campus. So I returned to Champaign-Urbana on June 10 and stayed home for a month. During that time I went into the office every day. I completed the first draft of my book manuscript, *Designing for Diversity*, and submitted it to the University of Illinois Press. I had been working on it for the past four years, and I desperately wanted to finish it before leaving for California.

Every noon hour I squeezed in a swim at a local swimmimg pool. By now I had come to view exercise not simply as a way to relieve the stress of Barry's illness. Nor was it just a way for me to keep in shape. In fact, it was much more than that. For me, exercise had taken on a quality that was almost spiritual. Every time I stepped outside for a walk or jumped into a swimming pool, I thought of all the days I had spent in the hospital with Barry. And I pictured all the patients stuck in bed at that moment, who couldn't go outdoors to exercise even if they wanted to. I was glad that at least today, I was not one of them. I owed it to myself to celebrate my good health. I also came to philosophize about something else: *that every day that Barry was not in the hospital was a good day.*

By the time I left Urbana on July 16, 1997, I had put all my administrative tasks in order, finished cleaning up my desk, said good-bye to my colleagues and friends, and prepared for my upcoming sabbatical. After my last seven years of teaching, I couldn't believe that I finally had some time off. By now I was ready for it.

When I said good-bye to 309 West Pennsylvania, I had no idea when I would return. I packed only a small suitcase with summer clothes. I pulled out the pages of my Day-Timer through October 1997, guessing that I would be back by then. My sabbatical leave was just for the fall term and I assumed that I would be back to teach in January. When I filled out the postal forms to forward our mail, on the space marked "Date of Return," I answered "???" Never had I taken a trip away from home before not knowing when I would return. It was an odd sensation.

In the meantime, Barry and I were on the phone just about every day. He was my last call of the night and my first call in the morning.

Shortly before I left for California he informed me that he had not been doing well.

"I seem to be bleeding again," he said. "I'm afraid that the tumor in my stomach may have returned."

"If you don't feel up to it, don't bother meeting me at the airport," I told him. "I'll look for you at the gate but if I don't see you, I'll take a shuttle back to the apartment. I'll assume you're either at the doctor's or at the hospital."

When I arrived and walked through the jet way at Lindbergh Field, I panned the crowd searching for his Greek fisherman's cap and black beard. But he wasn't there. My heart sped into high gear.

"Grab a taxi and dash straight over to Island Inn," I told myself. "Then call the hospital. He must be there. This trip is starting off on the wrong foot!"

As I raced towards the baggage claim Barry suddenly appeared. As usual he was running late. He looked pale and gaunt. When I gave him his usual bear hug, I could feel that his arms and shoulders were noticeably thinner and had lost much of their muscle mass. And with his new set of glasses, his face looked smaller to me. Later I could see that his legs, too, had shrunk. The illness was taking its toll on his body.

Barry later reflected on his deterioration.

> I first felt the cancer when Dr. Fromm in Detroit had Kathy, my mother, and me put our hands on my lower abdomen and we all sensed the belly cavity cancer. I would not have felt that on my own, and it was removed a day later.
>
> And it was not until the late summer of 1996 that I began feeling the cancer first in my abdomen wall, and then later in other parts of the abdomen, when the liver was beginning to protrude. I sensed that particularly when I was in the shower. Strangely though, Dr. Johnson, my oncologist at Carle Hospital in Urbana, never did tell me that she felt the cancer growing with her own hands. In fact, more often than not, she couldn't really feel much of anything. So after a while I stopped asking her.
>
> But around Thanksgiving 1996, my appetite began to diminish. I sensed well before the New Year that I was less

hungry, thinner, and had more protrusions than usual. It was in that state that I left for California.

None of this panicked me, though I was clearly concerned about it, perhaps because I strongly suspected that I would be coming out to San Diego and that something would be done, at least in the short run, to arrest my tumor growth...if all went well, of course.

My body changed more in late spring 1997. I was losing weight but my abdomen was sticking out even more. Plus I was losing strength. In April, my body still looked relatively normal to the average observer, provided I was fully clothed. But by June, one could easily tell that I had lost weight and that my shape was rather awkward.

As early as May, I could sense that I was losing weight in my shoulders. And when two friends came to see me in early June, and one of them gave me a hug, she said that she felt there was a whole lot less of me. Naturally that made me more self-conscious. Later I felt my legs were much thinner than ever before.

When I first noticed it, I was concerned, not alarmed. I wasn't happy about it but it did not keep me up at night. There was no point in panicking over something that I couldn't control all that much. I didn't realize how little I could control it until later.

Within hours of my arrival, we began a series of never-ending appointments with Dr. Jurgen Kogler, Barry's oncologist; Joy Hamer, the clinical oncology research nurse; Dr. Jeffrey Pressman, the gastroenterologist; and what seemed like a slew of other nurses and technicians. During these few weeks, Barry would undergo almost daily blood drawings, a CT-scan, a bone scan, two endoscopies, a colonoscopy, and an upper gastro-intestinal and small-bowel exam. After a while, we began to wonder whether there were any more medical tests left to administer. In order to raise his hemoglobin level, which had sunk into the low 7's, he received two additional units of blood, his first transfusions in almost two years.

With each test we dreaded the worst. Yet our fears were not realized. Much to our surprise, we discovered that Barry had a bleeding

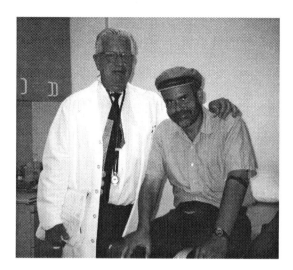

A later shot showing Barry and Dr. Jurgen Kogler, the oncologist who oversaw his treatment at Sharp Hospital and Clinic. San Diego, California; July 2000. (credit: author)

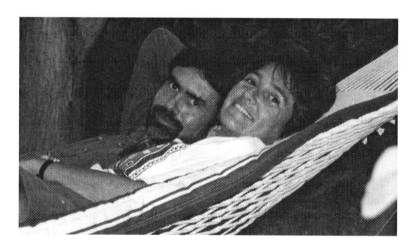

Relaxing on a hammock at my sister's house the day after my arrival in California. Because his hemoglobin level dropped quickly that day, Barry could not walk more than a few yards at a time. Irvine, California; July 1997. (credit: Mary Anne Anthony Smith)

ulcer, a condition that could be controlled by taking a pill called Prilosec. Just a few pills and his troubles would be over? That seemed almost too easy. But once Barry began taking them his bleeding ceased, and things slowly began to return to normal, even though his hemoglobin did not rise significantly.

In the midst of all this Barry was agonizing over whether or not to participate in his Mid-America history conference again this year. He had missed the conference twice before on account of his surgeries. This time the meeting was in Stillwater, Oklahoma, and Barry was slated to be a commentator on three papers. And he was tormented by another decision. Even though he had had his share of setbacks since he had been out in California, he felt an obligation to go back to work. He missed his job.

"Why can't I just commute from Urbana to San Diego on a weekly basis whenever I need the drug? I can do my teaching at Eastern in two or three days a week, and then travel cross-country for treatment. I'm sure I could do it." Barry said.

"Because it's crazy! It's ridiculous!" I said. "First of all it's expensive! CEOs and politicians may travel cross-country every week, but someone else is paying their travel expenses. We're not in that league. And second, it's dangerous! If something goes wrong in the meantime, you'll be dropped from the study. We both struggled to keep you in the Vitaxin protocol. Now don't set yourself up to be thrown right out of it! If staying in the protocol is one of your top priorities, you need to stay right here! Don't even think of leaving!"

We argued about this subject countless times that spring and summer, first over the phone and then in person. Each time I felt more and more frustrated. And I couldn't figure out why Barry was being so stubborn. Finally he snapped out of it.

That turned out to be a wise move, because in September the monster reappeared. For weeks when I woke up in the morning I had spotted a small growth on Barry's head near the tumor that had been excised just a few months ago. At first I thought it might just be a harmless trace of acne, but given his history, I doubted it could be that simple.

Finally, I confronted him. "Why don't you just keep your Greek fisherman's cap on whenever you see the doctor? If we hide what might prove to be any new evidence of cancer growth, you will probably be kept on the protocol."

Yet if we did nothing, the problem might get worse. If his head needed more treatment, it was better to have it sooner than later. We were in a Catch 22. But he insisted the doctor see it, and I watched as

Barry gingerly lifted his cap. I was hoping for the best but expecting the worst.

Dr. Kogler took one look at the spot and said, "It looks like it's back again."

Then he called in Dr. Y, the surgeon who had operated on Barry's head last spring. He took one look at it and said, "Yep. It's back."

"There's no point in operating again," Dr. Kogler said. "Look how fast it came back. You're probably best off trying radiation. I can recommend a good radiation oncologist right here in the building, Dr. Ronald Scott."

In an instant we were back where we were in April. Was Barry about to be ejected from the study once again? Could we possibly put ourselves through this spin cycle one more time? And deal with yet another doctor?

Unfortunately this latest crisis surfaced around my birthday. My 40th birthday had been marred by operation #3. Now for this, my 42nd, another thundercloud loomed overhead. Our friend, Dan Shaw—the one who had rescued Barry during his bleeding episode a few months earlier —had taken us to celebrate my birthday at the Boat House, one of my favorite restaurants on Harbor Island. After lunch Barry found a pay phone near the marina and called Dr. Gutheil, the Director of Clinical Oncology Research who was overseeing the protocol. He had asked Barry to call him sometime that day to follow up on this latest development. Dan and I watched as Barry, crouched next to the phone booth, spoke with the doctor at length. I was struck by the juxtaposition of Barry in the midst of his life-and-death conversation against the backdrop of the pleasure boats.

"It doesn't look good," Barry said when he returned. "It sounds as if I'm going to be dropped from the study —immediately. But I need to call back tomorrow to find out more."

I could feel another torpedo about to hit. And so could Barry.

> I was tempted to respond the way Willy Loman did when he was fired in *Death of a Salesman*: "A man is not a piece of fruit." Wisely, though, I held my tongue. Clearly, I don't have the kind of case that I had in the spring. For one, there's very little ambiguity in the protocol this time around. For another,

my cancer had grown since the last time. And finally, it looks as if the medical community and the biotech company are more or less in agreement now.

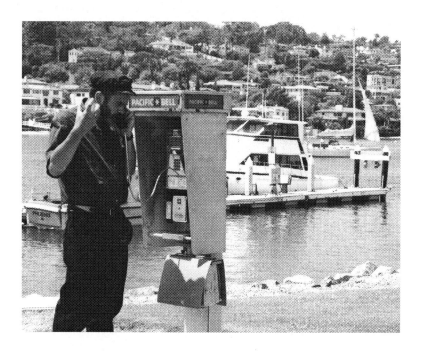

On several occasions Barry called Dr. John Gutheil, who was overseeing the Vitaxin protocol, to learn if he would be continued in the study. Many life and death discussions occurred at scenic phone booths such as this one in Shelter Island. San Diego, California; September 1997. (credit: author)

So on yet another day from the lobby of the historic Horton Grand Hotel, Barry phoned Dr. Gutheil.

The doctor told him, "Typically when there's a major growth of some kind anywhere in the body, that would be sufficient reason to terminate the participation in a protocol. But I can't say exactly what the biotechnology company will conclude."

On September 11 my Dad treated us for my birthday at The Grille, one of my favorite eateries in La Jolla. As we munched on bread and butter, we explained to Dad our medical events of the past few days. He could see that I was fighting to hold back the tears.

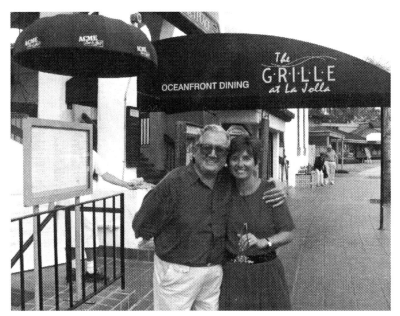

With my Dad, Harry Anthony, at the Grille celebrating my 42nd birthday. At the time we feared that Barry would be dropped from the Vitaxin protocol, with nowhere left to turn. La Jolla, California; September 1997. (credit: Barry Riccio)

The day after my birthday we had our first appointment with Dr. Scott, the radiation oncologist. After telling him where we were from, we had a pleasant surprise: we learned that he was a graduate of the University of Illinois. We instantly established a good rapport.

"Yes, I remember spending one winter there in particular, he told us. "I stepped into the Deluxe, a local eatery, and ate a hamburger there. When I walked in it was winter. Only an hour or so later it was summer. I had missed spring!"

"That's Champaign-Urbana, alright!" I said.

Dr. Scott seemed confident that he could eliminate the cancer on Barry's head and that it wouldn't return —at least in the same spot. He also stressed that Barry should not be dropped from the study.

"It's clear to me that your tumors have grown only along the scar line, an area that has very few blood vessels," Dr. Scott said. "Consequently, one would not expect the Vitaxin to have much effect in that region. In my view this is not a new growth. It's not a recurrence. It's the same cancer that you had back in April. The surgeon just didn't get it all."

"Could it also be that my head tumors started growing while I was off the Vitaxin last spring?" Barry asked. "During the debacle with the biotechnology company, I was denied treatment for almost three months."

"That's another very real possibility, especially since the drug seems to have been working so well for you," said Dr. Scott. "In any case, I'll be happy to make the case for you with your research team. You shouldn't be tossed out of the study just because of this."

After speaking with Dr. Scott, we both breathed a sigh of relief. It seemed that this new doctor was coming to our rescue. How lucky we were to have found him—and an Illini to boot!

But another conversation with Dr. Gutheil that same day muddied the waters further. It turns out that both he and the biotechnology company wanted to finish up Barry's current round of treatments and give him a CT-scan in another three weeks. That way they would have more data. He suggested that Barry hold off on radiation for another few weeks, as having the two treatments —the Vitaxin and the radiation —together would only confound the research findings.

Here is how Barry recalled this latest dilemma.

> Fair enough. But he also said that once I had the radiation I probably never could get back into the Vitaxin program. After all, the reason for doing the radiation in the first place would be that the tumors had spread, suggesting that the drug had not been all that effective, even if the cancer in my liver continued to be stable. Besides, if the tumor grew beyond the scar line, that would indicate that Vitaxin was ineffective even where blood vessels could transport the drug.
>
> To my mind it seemed irrational to let my head be taken care of by radiation and then be told because I had the problem there to begin with, nothing at all could be done about my liver, where I have made minimal progress. By the research doctor's own admission, I could be gone within months without the Vitaxin.... If all that sounds confusing, it's because it is, even to me.

All this happened when Barry would have been going out to Oklahoma for his conference. By now I had convinced him that traveling so far alone would have been unwise. He had sent his comments to his former office partner, Mark White, who read them on his behalf.

And suddenly one morning, we both came across a front-page article in *The Los Angeles Times* that made us stop in our tracks. It was about a Food and Drug Administration (FDA) Reform Bill that had just cleared the Senate with a vote of 98-2.

One sentence caught our attention: "Terminally ill cancer and AIDS patients already had the right to be treated off-protocol."

Off protocol? Could this be true? If so that could solve our dilemma. Barry needed radiation to treat the cancer on his head, but if he received the radiation he would be knocked off the protocol. Once again he was in a Catch 22. Why couldn't he get the Vitaxin *and* be treated off-protocol?

"Let's track down the reporter who wrote the story," I said. "Let's make sure we read it right. Maybe the reporter knows even more."

So Barry called *The LA Times* and left a detailed message explaining his situation. Within minutes the reporter returned his call, confirmed the story, and offered us some additional contacts. Barry followed up with phone calls to a few legislative assistants to Senator James Jeffords of Vermont, the sponsor of the bill that had just been passed. The next call was to the FDA to follow up with our contact there last spring. Once again we were getting our guns in order, just in case.

But within only a few days Barry's tumor on his head began to bleed non-stop. Again he was forced to wear that huge white bandage around his head. Now we had no time to waste. Something had to be done.

Finally, Dr. Gutheil and the biotechnology company reached a compromise. They agreed that Barry should proceed with the radiation treatments and then resume the Vitaxin. And Dr. Scott agreed to split the radiation into two different rounds in order to accommodate the research protocol. At least for the time being, we no longer had to be "on guard." While we had yet another respite, we began to wonder how long this one would last. Barry received radiation on his head throughout the month of October and then again in December, after he had finished his fourth round of Vitaxin. And much to the doctor's surprise, the radiation not only stopped the bleeding on Barry's head, but it also healed up the tumor much more quickly than he had expected.

"I think the combination of the radiation plus the Vitaxin must have done the trick," said Dr. Scott. "I've never seen radiation work so fast on a sarcoma before!"

As a result of the radiation, Barry was left with an even larger bald spot on his head. His operation that spring had left him with a spot about the size of a quarter. With the radiation came even greater hair loss. Now the bald spot had grown to the circumference of a large jar. According to Dr. Scott, the skin would be sensitive to sunlight for at least a year and a half, so he needed to keep it covered.

"A year and a half?" I wondered. "Would he even be around by then?"

As a result, his Greek fisherman's cap, which he had begun wearing last spring, now became a permanent fixture. It suited him well.

To relieve the tension of our medical mania, I escaped into the world of photography and enrolled in a one-day composition work-shop. Soon afterwards I invested in a tripod and traveled about the region shooting one scene after another. Barry joined me for all my expeditions and assisted with my new equipment. I even attempted night photography. I spent hours photographing the night time skyline, the historic architecture of Balboa Park, the cliffs at Torrey Pines State Beach, and the holiday lights at Hotel del Coronado.

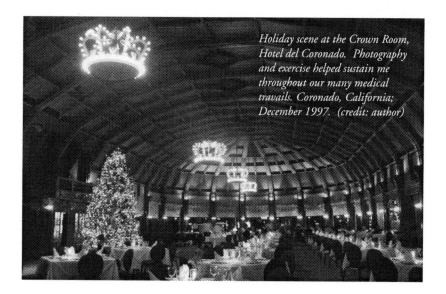

Holiday scene at the Crown Room, Hotel del Coronado. Photography and exercise helped sustain me throughout our many medical travails. Coronado, California; December 1997. (credit: author)

Our time in San Diego was punctuated by visitors. Over the span of several months, about 50 friends and relatives came to see us. Two sets of friends visited us ten times. My former research assistant flew down from the Bay Area, bringing Barry one of his favorite Bruce Springsteen tapes. Together we visited the San Diego Zoo, the Wild Animal Park, and Sea World. One weekend our friend, Dean, flew down from San Francisco, bringing Peter with him as a surprise. When they both appeared at our apartment door, Barry's face lit up. Later that day, Dan took us all out for a lovely sailboat ride.

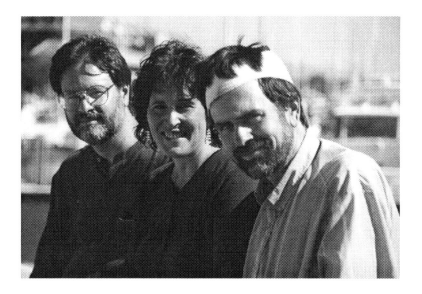

A bandaged Barry with his brother and sister-in-law, Greg and Maria Riccio, who visited from Arizona. Barry's head was bleeding once again, and he was about to begin radiation treatments. San Diego, California; October 1997. (credit: author)

Dan, Barry, and I went sailing several times that fall. I had taken lessons over 20 years ago on Mission Bay and was hooked on the sport ever since. The three of us even attempted the more ambitious San Diego Bay. With its cruise ships and naval carriers floating by, it was more of a challenge. It was the perfect way to spend a sabbatical.

We celebrated Barry's 43rd birthday at the Reuben E. Lee, a replica of a Mississippi riverboat docked at the edge of Harbor Island. Our

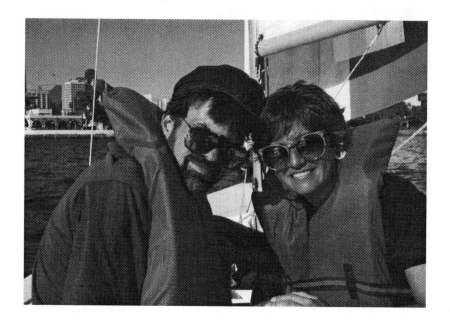

Sailing on San Diego Bay, terrific medicine for both of us. San Diego, California; October 1997. (credit: Daniel Shaw)

wedding reception was held there in 1980. We reminisced about Barry's last several birthday celebrations with friends in Urbana. This time only Felicia joined us. Once again I wondered if this would be Barry's final birthday. At the same time, I was thrilled that he had made it this far. Had he stayed in Urbana, he might have been gone by now.

That fall, Casey and Mary arrived from Flagstaff. They were the couple who had thrown the fabulous tenure party for Barry. Since we had last seen them they had moved from Illinois to Arizona, and they drove nine hours just to see Barry. It was exhilarating to see our Midwestern friends in a new setting. And Barry was pleased with how his friends found him.

As he put it, "Casey thought I showed a considerable amount of energy, even though my hemoglobin level was considerably low at the time, and I was still losing weight."

In the midst of Barry's many medical appointments, we squeezed in a few days away. We took a scenic two-day trip to Santa Barbara with Mary.

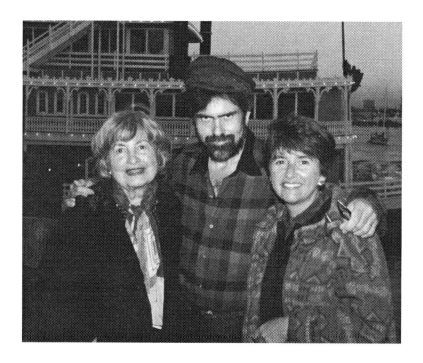

Celebrating Barry's 43rd birthday with his mother, Felicia Riccio, at the Reuben E. Lee on Harbor Island. Our wedding reception was held there in 1980. San Diego, California; November 1997. (credit: author)

We spent the evening of Halloween at my sister's house in Irvine. It was the first time I had ever seen my nieces decked out in costumes, and we enjoyed watching all the trick-or-treaters stop at One Caraway. Earlier that day, we visited two friends who treated us to a lavish Indian buffet lunch. I had been anxious to spend Halloween at a real house. More than any other day of the year, I missed our house in Urbana. Just thinking about it gave me pangs of pain. A few weeks before, the bright yellow leaves on our maple trees would have been at their peak. It was the first autumn I wouldn't see them.

But it wasn't only Halloween that triggered my memories of home. Sometimes I would lie awake in our Island Inn bed early in the morning and pretend that I was in our bedroom in Urbana watching the sun shine into our Palladian window. I couldn't help but wonder what must have been spinning around in our house's mind while we were away.

"Where was Barry? Why wasn't he coming back?," it would have been thinking last spring. "His clothes are hanging in the closets, his books are filling the shelves, but he's not here. This place feels different without him."

And this fall, even more confusion, "And where did Kathy go? Why isn't she coming back? She planted all those purple petunias in our window boxes in June, and then she went away. Her car is still in the garage, and her stuff is all over the house. Even the mailman doesn't come by here any more. I took good care of those two for the past 12 years. Now, they've abandoned me!"

Whenever I had these thoughts, a wave of guilt would sweep through me. It was almost as if I had left a pet home alone for months, anxiously awaiting the return of her master. Ironically, the more time I spent at Island Inn, the more these feelings subsided—and the more our tiny apartment began to feel like home.

As the weeks rolled by, I often wondered what would happen after the holidays when my sabbatical leave was up and it was time for me to return home. As long as Barry remained on the Vitaxin protocol, he had to remain in California. The drug was brand new, it was only in a phase one trial, and it hadn't yet been approved by the Food and Drug Administration. He could only get it in San Diego. But did I need to stay here with him too? By October it was already time to arrange my teaching schedule for the upcoming spring semester.

"Yes, I am planning to return," I told my colleagues at Illinois. "Go ahead and schedule my two courses in the Spring Semester Timetable."

At the time I believed I would be back. No other option was even waiting in the wings.

But would Barry be back with me? Just the thought of leaving him behind turned my stomach inside out. He had already had enough health problems while I was with him. Who knows what might happen if I were to leave? Images of Barry at his worst swirled around my head. April: the aftermath of his scalp operation, his head totally wrapped up like a mummy in the ugly, flesh-colored bandage. Blood dripping down from the skin graft on his leg and onto our carpet. September: the reappearance of his scalp tumor, with a huge white bandage strapped around his head like a prisoner of war. All the while, the prospect of being tossed out of the protocol—thrown away like a piece of meat — loomed overhead. How could he handle another episode alone? And from afar, how could I?

Yet if he were no longer on the Vitaxin study, and nothing else could be done for him out here, we had little choice but to return home. After all that we'd been through in the meantime —the hype and the hope —how would it feel to arrive back home? We couldn't fool ourselves. Barry would be going home to die.

Every time I turned the page on our calendar, I could see that my date of departure was drawing closer and closer. Halloween pumpkins gave way to Thanksgiving turkeys. Then one day I walked into a store, and there he was: that fat man with a bright red suit and furry hat, perched high up in his sleigh. I used to love that sight, a sign that Christmas vacation was only a few weeks away. But this time was different.

"No, not now. It's just too soon," I thought. "I'm not ready to leave. Not yet."

And every time I saw another wreath, another Christmas tree, or another fake snowflake, those words echoed in my mind. After some soul-searching in November I wrote my colleagues that it was possible I might not return in January.

"Depending upon Barry's situation," I said, "I might need to stay out with him longer and extend my leave. But I won't know for sure until the end of December when he will have his next set of CT-scans."

As I wrote this message a surge of guilt swept through me. Replacing a faculty member at the last minute is not easy. I could feel that tug of war between my professional and personal lives. Ever since Barry had become ill, I felt yanked between those two worlds. For over four years, while Barry was in the hospital and we were off on our many medical trips, I had already taken scores of sick leave days. Each time I left my teaching duties behind. Could I abandon them once more? *Was I a professor first, a wife second? Or the other way around?* Every time I thought about it, my stomach turned in knots.

But when sabbatical would be over, my salary would be too. If I stayed in San Diego with Barry, how would we survive financially? One day in late November, my parents came to the rescue. I explained the turmoil I was going through.

"If you need help, just ask," they said. "We can help tide you over for a few more months."

"What a relief," I thought. "I'll be very grateful."

How I wish they had told me this earlier. It would have spared me weeks of anguish. At least now I had a backup plan, just in case. Nonetheless I had mixed feelings about taking money from my parents. After being financially independent for 20 years, it felt like a giant leap backwards. I felt a tinge of guilt, embarrassment, and shame. But after a while, I talked myself out of it. I decided that if I was lucky enough to have parents who could help us, refusing their offer would be insane.

Barry, too, reluctantly asked his mother for money. Until this point, even though he had been battling this illness for four years, he had been too proud to ask for help. Yet now, at my insistence, he did. It was the first time in our marriage that my own salary would be coming to a halt, and now he had no choice.

But the stress of our financial woes paled in comparison to the unpredictable rate of Barry's health. So we were both on pins and needles on Christmas Eve 1997 when we met with Dr. Kogler to learn the results of Barry's latest CT-scans. If they showed that the cancer had grown, then we'd need to start packing our bags and drive home. But if the cancer had been held in check yet again, then Barry would be approved for at least one more round of Vitaxin. And now I knew that I could stay on with him.

After giving Barry his routine physical exam, Dr. Kogler seemed ready to leave the room.

"What about the CT-scan?" we asked.

"Oh yes, that's right. Let me check into it. I'll be back in a few minutes," he said.

"Just remember, it's Christmas Eve," I said. "You're only allowed to deliver good news today."

Shortly afterwards, he returned.

"No change," he said. "The scans look basically the same as last time."

This was just the news we were hoping to hear. I gave Barry a "high-five." My months of turmoil were over. My gut-wrenching decision was now made for me. We would both stay on. When we drove home from the doctor's office that Christmas Eve, the holiday lights never looked brighter. It was going to be a merry Christmas.

CHAPTER SIX

Publicity and its Perils
(1997-1998)

"ONLY WHEN IT IS TRULY DARK CAN ONE REALLY SEE THE STARS."
— CHARLES BEARD

Much to our surprise, the view outside our tiny Island Inn apartment was often festive. Right after Thanksgiving a giant neon Christmas tree spanned the two Marriott Towers, and the top of the Hyatt was lit in red and green. During the January 1998 Superbowl, we could see two neon-lit helmeted players tossing a football back and forth above the San Diego Convention Center. During the summertime, we could see fireworks two to three times a week, the grand finale to various conventions. Whenever I heard them I ran to look out our window. Brilliant blues, purples, and reds exploded before my eyes, like a series of giant neon palm trees bursting open. No matter what had happened earlier that day, the fireworks always brightened our spirits.

Only a five-minute walk away, the boats in the Marriott Marina flashed their holiday displays. We took several evening walks along the harbor just to see them. No matter where we lived, I always loved driving around town to see Christmas decorations.

In the meantime, we both kept busy writing. Barry was reading steadily, diligently scribbling notes preparing for his second book, an upper level text on contemporary America since the 1970's. He had already written several essays that would eventually be folded into the book, including one on Operation Desert Storm, another on Clinton's health care proposal, and still another on Reagan's Tax Reform Act of 1986. But he had much more to do. He was first awarded the book contract back in March 1997 at the behest of his office partner, Mark. At the time, I hesitated to see him take on another obligation knowing that his health might not hold up in time to finish it. Yet in retrospect, it turned out to be a wise decision. For Barry, reading history was recreation. No matter if he was pouring over the pages of *Turmoil and Triumph, John Wayne's America*, or *Liberalism and its Discontents*, he was off in another world. Barry had always been an avid reader. While he was immersed in his teaching over the past several years, he often wished he had more time to read through the thousands of books in his personal library. Ironically, most of his books were still sitting on our bookshelves in Urbana while he was thousands of miles away. Eventually I sent out a few more boxes of books for him. Now, he finally had time for what he enjoyed most: reading. On occasion, he would notice that one of the plays he had just read was being performed locally, so we would get tickets to see it. For both of us the performing arts had become an escape from our own day-to-day drama.

And I was busy revising *Designing for Diversity*, what now had become my 400-page magnum opus. It had become overwhelming, and I was anxious to finish it up and move onto other things. But the revision process was painstakingly slow. On cloudy days I had no difficulty working on the project. But when the sun beckoned I had a hard time. I couldn't help but think about the bitter cold and winter winds I was missing back home. When the rest of the world was freezing I was basking in 60 and 70 degree weather. Barry could have easily worked all day long no matter what the weather, but I could not. For him, the novelty of our new environment seemed to have worn off, even though he never stopped loving San Diego. But for me, our days in Southern California were numbered. Who knew how much longer I would be able to enjoy this beautiful place? And who knew how much more "quality time" we would have together? I decided that the work could wait. So, after a few hours of writing each day, I closed up my files, turned off the computer, and went outside for a walk with Barry. It turned out to be an ideal work schedule.

Even though I was relieved to stay in San Diego with Barry, after a while the drawbacks of our tiny apartment began to surface. Island Inn was designed primarily to house low-to moderate-income tenants for short-term stays. Given Barry's disability paycheck from the State of Illinois, he qualified. Ironically, even his $38,000 annual faculty salary from Eastern Illinois University qualified him as a low-to-moderate income resident in San Diego! By contrast, I saw myself as a visitor. I hesitated to receive mail in the building. Instead I had it forwarded to my parents' house, where I would pick it up a couple times a week. I hesitated to tell casual acquaintances where we lived, since I feared that, given that I was living here with Barry, putting him over the income limit, we might be evicted. Oddly enough months later, when my income from the university had stopped, I qualified as low-to moderate-income myself. And having lived at Island Inn for over several months, my status as a visitor was questionable.

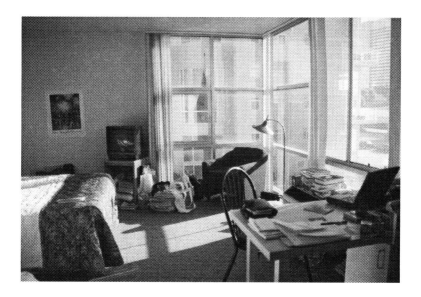

Stacks of books, files, and clothes filled our tiny but bright studio apartment at Island Inn. Within months we could barely see the floor. San Diego, California; November 1997. (credit: author)

Because I saw our living quarters as only temporary, I hesitated to purchase any household items. For almost a year Barry lived with a stark, institutional decor, but eventually I caved in. At a snail's pace, our hotel room was transformed into an apartment. The first item to go up on the walls was a free poster from the San Diego Convention and Visitors' Bureau, a colorful image of fireworks over the skyline. Months later, I taped up two free posters from the Sidney Kimmel Cancer Center. Later I shelled out $10 on a poster of a tropical beach scene. It took several months before I replaced the ugly floral bedspread stained with cigarette burns. And that was only because my cousins had commented on how dreary it looked. Soon afterwards, I invested in a set of jade plaid sheets to replace the plain white ones that the hotel provided. But we held onto the receipt and didn't open the package until after Barry's next CT-scan. If his test results had looked bad, we'd say good-bye to our new decor and ask for a refund. It took me several more months to fork out $4 a piece for a set of black plastic crates. That helped us finally make a small dent in the piles of books and clothes spread all over the floor.

The least glamorous aspect of Island Inn was the size of our apartment. Our unit was only 300 square feet, including a sleeping area, a small kitchenette, and a private bath. It was more like a motel room than an apartment. For just a few days or weeks, it was fine. But after several months the cramped quarters—with all our worldly goods piled all over the floor—sometimes got on my nerves. I was all the more troubled whenever I thought of us paying for our nine-room house in Urbana to sit empty.

While we owned a house full of furniture in the Midwest, at Island Inn we had only a queen-sized bed, a dresser with three drawers and a lamp, a TV on a stand, one comfortable reading chair covered with blue fabric, and one uncomfortable chair with a black vinyl seat. Attached to the kitchen cabinets was a 2' x 4' surface that doubled as our kitchen table, as our bill-paying headquarters, and as our workspace for our laptop computer, portable printer, and office supplies. It was a tight squeeze. Only one of us fit at the table, and that was pushing it. At times I had to avoid splashing droplets of squash soup on my computer disks. In the meantime, Barry ate in the blue chair or on the bed, precariously balancing a plate on his lap and a drink on the floor.

Due to our severe space shortage, several items that would normally be stored in our apartment lived like stowaways in the trunk of our car. At times I felt like a gypsy on wheels. We were usually driving around with an odd assortment of beach chairs, towels, a tripod, a pair of tennis shoes and socks, jackets and sweaters, as well as a borrowed raincoat.

The kitchenette was attractive, with white particleboard cabinets, a small microwave oven, and a pint-sized refrigerator such as you would find in a student dorm room. I could barely cram four small frozen dinners in the freezer, but that was pushing it. The refrigerator had only four small shelves, forcing us to visit the grocery store several times a week. We could only buy food that fit on the pullout basket of the grocery cart, because otherwise it would not fit in our refrigerator.

What was missing from our apartment? A couch, for one. We became experts at musical chairs, rotating from the blue chair to the black chair to the bed. We lacked a stove and oven as well, so we were unable to do any serious cooking. With the exception of a small medicine cabinet, the bathroom lacked storage space. My cosmetics bag resided on the tiny kitchen counter, where at times my toothbrush and contact lens case were only inches away from a bowl of piping hot tomato sauce. My hair dryer lived on the floor in one of my hiking boots. My umbrella lived in the other.

Within months both of our possessions spread out all over the floor. Our book writing generated its own clutter. Despite my best efforts to keep the place orderly, it soon became a mess. In Urbana, I had my study at home as well as two spacious offices at school. At Island Inn, I had nowhere else to write but our one and only room, rotating between the kitchen desk and the blue chair. My notes were scattered all over the place. Barry had never been a neatnick, far from it. But I was never messy by nature, so for me this transition was not easy.

But whenever I started feeling sorry for myself, I looked out our window and thought of all the homeless people who lived only blocks away. Until only recently, they had been the only residents of the Gaslamp Quarter. For a few days, a young Mexican woman, bundled up in an Indian blanket and carrying a bunch of plastic bags, made her home on the sidewalk. She staked out a spot diagonally across from Island Inn, next to a parking lot and in front of an abandoned ware-house. Late at night, while peering through the vertical blinds, I could see her perched at the doorway. The next morning, she was still there. A few days later when it started raining, my heart ached for her.

"Quit complaining about two people being stuck in one room for over half a year!" I told myself. "That could be you out there. Compared to her, you're living in Buckingham Palace!"

Despite all this, in most other respects the place was ideal for us. We lived in two-month increments, never knowing how much longer we would stay. Signing a lease at another apartment building would have been impossible. Plus the rent for almost any nearby apartment was well over triple what we were paying. Without Island Inn, I have no idea where we would have gone. Had we been in most other cities, where such state-of-the-art temporary housing is almost non-existent, we would have been at a loss.

Adjacent to Children's Hospital at the Sharp Hospital and Clinic is an attractive Ronald McDonald House. Once I knocked on the door and took a self-guided tour. With its cathedral ceilings and sunshine streaming in the windows, it was striking. But it was designed to accommodate families whose children have serious illnesses, not for adults. And unlike MD Anderson there was no Rotary House in sight. Even if there had been, the cost of such a long-term stay would have been prohibitive. So for us, Island Inn was a lifeboat.

The staff at Island Inn was extremely efficient, and the building was unusually well managed. The receptionists at the front desk were friendly and accommodating not only to us, but also to our many visitors. Having guests stay at Island Inn was a windfall. At the time, rooms rented for only $38 a night, a fraction of what they were almost anywhere else in the city. And compared to hosting all our guests at home, it was actually much easier for me. With no sheets or towels to wash, no extra grocery shopping to do, and no meals to prepare or clean up after, I had enough energy to enjoy everyone's company.

Our apartment overlooked the entrance to the parking garage. We often heard radios blaring. A dark blue Chevy emitted reggae music. A cool black sports car sent off smooth jazz. And a black convertible, with its top wide open, played soaring arias from the opera. At first all this noise woke me up, but after a while I tuned it out.

But the worst sound of all was the street sweeper. It drove by every Monday and Friday at 2:30 a.m. The engine noise was piercing, awakening me from a deep sleep. Just when I managed to fall back into Never-Never land, the lion roared once more. The truck was now making its way back on the other side of the street. I never did get used to this ear-splitting screech.

In an effort to keep our expenses under control, we sought out discounts wherever we could. Every Thursday morning we picked up a copy of the *San Diego Reader*. As soon as I opened it I raced to the restaurant section where I clipped half-price coupons. We bought batches of five tickets at a time at a local movie theater. Through Arts Tix, we bought half-price tickets for same-day shows at local performing arts centers. In fact, seeing a play often cost us less than a movie. The local *Entertainment* book offered two-for-one coupons to a myriad of eateries, museums, and attractions all around town, and we used it religiously.

Had the climate been any different, we might have found Island Inn claustrophobic. And at times it was. During the El Niño storms of 1998 I often felt trapped inside our 300 square foot apartment. Yet fortunately, most days in San Diego were temperate, enabling us to spend a good chunk of our time outside.

Since we lacked much private space of our own, we adopted a number of public places as outdoor "living rooms." It reminded me of living in Europe, where tiny apartments force city-dwellers out to public plazas. Seagrove Park at Del Mar, the beaches and parks of La Jolla, the cliffs at Pacific Beach, and Fanuel Street Park at Mission Bay were among our favorites. So were Shelter Island and Harbor Island. At each of these locales, we would set up our two pink folding chairs, read for an hour or two, and then walk for miles along the waterfront trails.

On weekends we would drive to Balboa Park, only a few miles away. We discovered free walking tours around the park on Saturday mornings. Barry and I became students of the exotic palms and eucalyptus trees and learned about the history of the Spanish Colonial architecture along the Prado. The tours gave us a fresh set of lenses from which to view the city.

During the evenings, we adopted several indoor spots as our living rooms. The Victorian lobby of the Horton Grand Hotel, diagonally across the street, was one of them. We often went there for a cup of tea and to listen to live music. We became friendly with one of the pianists there and sometimes followed him to the Nordstrom department store, where he played jazz by the escalator. Another of our living rooms was Mimmo's Italian Village, where we heard live Italian opera and Spanish folk songs. We enjoyed listening to their renditions of "Feniculi, Fenicula," "Granada," and "Toreador" while eating our linguini with red clam sauce and sipping our Oranginas. Almost always, other musicians darted out of their chairs and started singing. Among them were an elderly Filipino man and a fellow who performed Russian dances. Another gentleman always sang "Oh What a Beautiful Morning" from *Oklahoma*. A woman in her 80's named Elizabeth, dressed in a floor-length gown, accompanied the pianist. For about $5 each, we had a delicious dinner and live entertainment. No doubt it was one of the city's best kept secrets.

Music became an important part of our new world. On weekends we would saunter over to the East Plaza Gazebo at Seaport Village to listen to live entertainment. Whether it was the jazz, soul, or disco we always left feeling upbeat. During the summer we sat out on our beach chairs at the Cove, where we enjoyed the La Jolla Concerts by the Sea. There the Mar Dels were among my favorites. At the San Diego Museum of Art's outdoor sculpture garden we heard a guitarist perform classical and contemporary variations of Baroque, Japanese, and Spanish music. At Navy Pier we discovered the San Diego Symphony Summer Pops. The stage jutted out into the bay, overlooking the harbor with its fluttering lights. Around sunset sailboats would glide by. At the end of each performance, a wonderful display of fireworks was set to music. For several hours, the music of the Pops, along with the stunning pyrotechnics, made our troubles vanish.

So despite our circumstances, every day I woke up thinking how grateful I was to be living—albeit temporarily—in such an uplifting environment. For Barry, too, San Diego was a delight. Almost every day, the sun was shining and the daily highs hovered between 65 and 75 degrees. The weather was absolutely perfect. All through the year, we could see leaves on the trees and flowers in bloom. While our impatiens at home were dead by mid-October, here we saw huge shrubs of impatiens all year round. The birds of paradise, the hibiscus, and the bouginvillias were all brilliant.

We routinely walked the streets of the Gaslamp Quarter. With 16

square blocks on the National Register for Historic Places, it had just
undergone a renaissance. It was now full of boutiques, restaurants, cafes,
and jazz bars. We admired its Victorian architecture and active street
life, which was hopping almost all night long. Any stroll down Fifth
Avenue was a stimulant to all five senses. Garlic aromas filled the air
from La Strada, Bella Luna, and Panevino, while the scent of ginger
emanated from the Royal Thai and the King and I. We walked along
miles of panoramic waterfront trails near Seaport Village and the two
Embarcadero Marina Parks. On the way we would pass the Convention
Center and the Marriott Hotel and watch the crowds pour onto the
streets. Each group of conventioneers temporarily took over downtown. With their identical conference badges, briefcases, and canvas
bags, you couldn't miss them. We strolled the arcades of Horton Plaza, a
downtown postmodern shopping and entertainment center painted in
wild golds, oranges, blues, and greens. There we would make weekly
trips to Long's Drugs for Barry's many prescriptions, and soon the staff
recognized us by name. One of our most frequent destinations was
Ralph's, a grocery store, only two blocks away. It was an award-winning
design with underground parking and a sidewalk cafe on its north and
west sides, a far cry from the typical sprawling grocery stores of the
suburbs. Nine times out of 10 we did our grocery shopping on foot,
European style.

And for me, having my parents only 12 miles up the road was
another stroke of luck. Mom cooked countless lunches for us, and she
and Dad hosted us regularly. Whether it was avgolemno soup, Greek
style chicken with rice, or Chinese vegetables, every meal there was a
delight. If I had time, I often sneaked in a swim and Jacuzzi at their
neighborhood pool. It was a treat for me to spend some time at a real
house, a welcome change from our small studio apartment.

Later my parents would join the local YMCA, and so did I. Every
morning I got into a new routine, driving 15 minutes up I-5 to meet
them for an hour-long workout.

Sometimes I purposely would take out my appointment book only
to compare the previous months with the current ones. While I was on
campus working, my calendar was always jam-packed. I could still
picture myself dashing from one office to the other, one meeting to
another, and one class to another. Yet now, apart from Barry's many

medical appointments, my time was my own. In an odd way, perhaps I had to wait for my calendar to clear so that that my head could, too. For both of us, it was like an early retirement.

This was what a leave was meant to be, the simple gift that anyone who works needs most: time. After four years of Barry's illness, I had finally come to the realization that no matter how hard I wished, we would never get our normal lives back. But at least, for the moment, I had time. That was no small matter. And I decided to try to live in what psychologists call "the here and now." Seize the day. Carpe diem. Don't worry about what tomorrow will bring.

———————

In late February we met with Dr. Gutheil.

"By the way, are you writing up anything about the Vitaxin research?" I asked him.

"In fact, just recently I sent off an abstract to ASCO, the American Society of Clinical Oncologists, conference. It's going to be held in Los Angeles later this spring. Would you like to see a copy of the abstract?"

"Yes, of course," I said. "We'll find it very interesting, I'm sure."

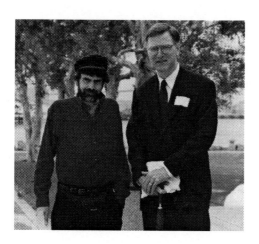

At the Cancer Survivors' March and Rally with Dr. John Gutheil of the Sidney Kimmel Cancer Center, who oversaw the Vitaxin protocol. In his speech that day, Dr. Gutheil stressed that more patients need to participate in clinical trials. San Diego, California; September 1998. (credit: author)

"So Barry, how are you feeling?" he asked.

"My energy level is good, and I'm still walking about two to four miles a day. Last week I hiked three days in a row in the desert near Palm Springs. Some of the trails were uphill, with fairly steep grades," said Barry.

"Terrific," the doctor said. "How's your weight?"

"It's actually up a few pounds," Barry replied. "I'm about 172 now."

"Good. Do you have any pain?"

"Yes, from time to time. I've had occasional discomfort in my abdomen, but not much. But most of the time, I've felt fine."

"Let's take a look at your head," Dr. Gutheil said.

Barry slowly removed his Greek fisherman's cap.

"It's healing up well," the doctor said. "The scar looks good."

"What's happening with the Vitaxin study? How soon will Phase two be ready?" Barry asked.

"It's being held up at the moment. But none of that should have any impact on your situation. You 'come on the cheap' since you have only the minimal dosage (.1) of the drug, especially compared to the latest patients who had much more than that amount. At this point there's no problem with your being retreated," Dr. Gutheil replied.

"What about the others on the phase one study? How have they done so far?" Barry asked.

"Out of the 15 patients in phase one, only two people have been retreated, you and another woman. She went through three or four cycles. The others either had to drop out of the study, or their cancer progressed more than 25%, so after the first round of the protocol, they were discontinued. But don't worry. You're doing well. In fact, you're way out there."

"It's hard to believe that it's already February, and Barry has now been on the Vitaxin for just over a year," I added. "I know that doctors are always cautious, but at least to me, it sure looks as if this drug is working. What do you think?"

"I would say that at this point, yes, it appears to be," said Dr. Gutheil. "But we don't know why."

As we left SKCC we felt exhilarated. One year after Barry had made his journey west, he was still here. Who ever could have imagined that? And the tumors in his liver, which were roaring out of control when he left Illinois, had continued to stabilize. He had made it only by the skin of his teeth.

Instead of heading straight back to Island Inn, I made a detour to the Torrey Pines Gliderport to take advantage of the remaining minutes of daylight. A few paragliders were soaring over the cliffs, while a lone hangglider was making its descent. Gusty winds almost blew Barry's Greek fisherman's cap off his head. After hiking down a small trail, we could see a spectacular panorama. The ocean was navy blue and churning with whitecaps. Ominous clouds loomed over the horizon, yet the sun's rays were bursting through. The coast of La Jolla was off to our south, and Torrey Pines State Beach and Del Mar were off to our north.

"You did it, Barry! I can't believe it! It's almost too good to be true! Congratulations!" I told him.

Our latest two-month drama was over, and the next one was about to begin.

Within 24 hours, I was on a plane headed back to the Midwest. Several events drew me back home. Our School of Architecture was undergoing its five-year accreditation process. The Women's Studies Program at the University of Chicago had invited me to give a lecture. And I was slated to give a presentation at the Environmental Design Research Association (EDRA) conference in St. Louis. Like Barry's Mid-America Conference, EDRA was the event that I had attended religiously until he got sick. After that, I had missed several years in a row, so I was anxious to get back.

And most importantly, it was tax time. I needed to review all our financial papers, half of which were in San Diego and half of which were filed away at home. I had scheduled an appointment with our tax preparer several weeks in advance of my trip.

This was the first stretch where Barry had been doing well enough that I felt comfortable leaving him alone. Mom and Dad had reassured me that if anything went wrong, he could call on them. And Felicia would be coming out to spend part of that time with him too. I was planning to be away for three weeks.

As my plane made its descent into Willard Airport, rows and rows of brown cornfields came into view. I was overwhelmed with the vast nature of the prairie, just as I had been almost 14 years ago when I had first flown into Champaign. When we first moved to Illinois the prairie landscape seemed so odd to me, and the Mediterranean scenery of California was where I felt most at home. Yet over the years the pattern reversed itself. Whenever I flew back into Willard, more and more, it felt like home, while whenever I had flown back out to California, it felt less so. But now, after only seven months' absence, I was back where I started. What had long been familiar now seemed unfamiliar. Once again I was struck by the flat, desolate prairie. It was the longest I had ever been away from Urbana.

Our house sitter was waiting for me at the airport and drove me home. It was an unusually warm day for February. The Midwest had experienced a mild winter, an apparent side effect of El Niño. When we drove up the driveway to 309 West Pennsylvania, our bright white trellis, shutters, and railings all stood out to greet me. They were happy to have me back.

The day after my talk at the University of Chicago, I was back on the Amtrak headed south to St. Louis for the EDRA conference. Over the next several days I reacquainted myself with several colleagues from around the country. I enjoyed being back in the academic swing of things.

Nonetheless, when I returned to Champaign, reality set in. At home my tax preparations kept me up until 2 a.m. several nights in a row.

At my office at 412 Architecture, I found twenty huge boxes piled all over the floor. It looked as if a family of four had just moved in. During my absence, my two offices were combined into one, since my administrative post had ended. One by one, I started opening the boxes. I would arrive at the office first thing in the morning and stay there until after 11:00 at night. I was overwhelmed, and decided that I needed to extend my stay for another three weeks.

Ironically, it was not until the day that I left town that I could actually see the floor in 412 Architecture again.

———— • ◆ • ————

In the meantime, that March Dr. Gutheil organized an international conference on monoclonal antibodies. He invited Barry to participate. When Barry called me to tell me about it, I was ecstatic. What a great opportunity to learn about the scientific research in which Barry was a guinea pig.

During the event, attended by some 400 participants, one of the plenary speakers was David Cheresh, a molecular and cell biologist from nearby Scripps Research Institute. His name was already familiar to us from *The New York Times* and *The San Diego Union-Tribune* stories several years ago, but this was the first time that Barry had actually seen him. More significantly, over a decade ago, he invented Barry's drug, Vitaxin. Barry watched in awe as Dr. Cheresh's presentation ended with a large graph flashed on the screen. It depicted the progress of one patient who had been on the Vitaxin treatment for over a year. Barry immediately recognized the graph as his own case.

"I felt like telling the stranger next to me, 'That's me!' but I held my tongue," Barry said.

Following the presentation, Dr. Gutheil introduced Barry to Dr. Cheresh, and the two joined each other with a group for lunch. David invited Barry to tour his lab at Scripps to see how his new drug was developed and to learn about his current research. The two of us took him up on his offer in April. Later that year, we joined him on his sailboat, Sorceress, on San Diego Bay. David guided us through his lab for two hours, and he introduced us to several colleagues. We saw the blood vessels of chick embryos, similar to those in humans. One of the computerized images enlarged the blood vessel 65,000 times so that they could be seen more clearly. It was a window into the world of science and computer technology that we had never seen before.

"I've been working on this type of research for a long time," David told us, "but if you were to have told me 10 years ago that today, I'd be sitting across the table from someone who has actually benefited from Vitaxin, I wouldn't have believed you. It's the first time that's happened to me. Some of us must wait a lifetime for this moment. And for some scientists, it never happens."

"That's so exciting!" I told him. "And whoever would have thought that we would be sitting across the table from someone who developed a treatment that would prolong Barry's life. What could we possibly do to help you and your research?"

"Let me think about it," he said. "I have an idea. I have a contact at *Time* magazine who had written about our research years ago. She'll probably be very interested in Barry's progress. Her name is Christine Gorman," as he leafed through his Rolodex. "Here's her phone number. Why don't you give her a call sometime?"

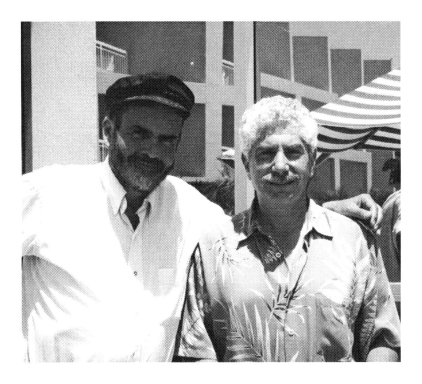

Barry with Dr. David Cheresh of the Scripps Research Institute, inventor of the antiantiogenic drug, Vitaxin, that prolonged Barry's life. La Jolla, California; August 2000. (credit: author)

Time magazine! The thought that *Time* magazine would find Barry's story of interest had never even crossed my mind. But it was certainly worth a try. We noted the information, but decided not to follow up right then. Instead we preferred to wait and see what the results of Barry's latest CT-scans would show. Deep down, I was afraid of doing anything that might jinx our success.

At about 10 a.m. on May 4, 1998, our phone rang. Out of the blue, a woman asked Barry for an interview about Vitaxin for the ABC Evening News that same night. That call started a wave of publicity that would besiege us all week. We can only speculate about what would have happened had we not been home that morning. Would Barry have remained an unknown?

Within minutes it seemed as if our phone would never stop ringing. Barry could barely hang up before it rang once again. A steady stream of messages backed up on our voice mail. The story had already snowballed.

We had planned to spend that week at a friend's cottage in Laguna Beach. This was also one of those rare weeks when Barry did not have any medical treatments and we could both travel out of town.

But our plans for a quiet week near the beach never did come to fruition. While we did drive up to Laguna right after the ABC interview, we spent much of our time checking our voice mail and returning phone calls. My job was to serve as Barry's agent, screening his calls and noting the contact information, and then sending out e-mail messages chronicling Barry's case to various journalists. Barry, meanwhile, spent several hours on the phone being interviewed just about every day. It seemed as if we couldn't get out the door before we had yet another voice mail message, another journalist wanting an interview.

That Monday the television crew from ABC Evening News invaded our tiny San Diego studio apartment. It took us over an hour to undo the damage after they left, removing piles of suitcases and clothes from our bed and rearranging stacks of books that had been knocked over on the floor. The place looked as if a tornado had just blown through. We soon decided that the next interview, if there were one at all, would be conducted elsewhere.

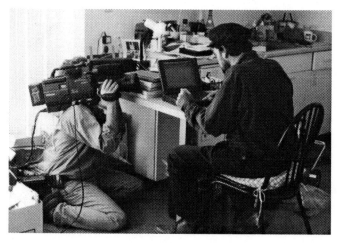

Barry with camera crew from ABC Evening News at our studio apartment. Within hours he went from obscurity to celebrity status. San Diego, California; May 1998. (credit: Gary Whitmer)

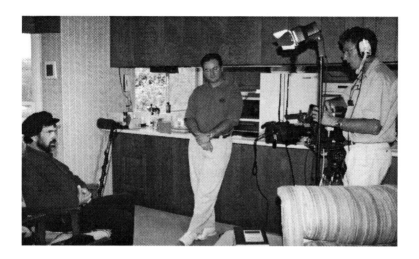

NBC Nightly News filming Barry at the home of my aunt and uncle, Helen and Joe Boltinghouse. By now our phone was ringing off the hook with reporters wanting to interview Barry. Whittier, California; May 1998. (credit: author)

Nevertheless, as Barry and I shut the door to #380 behind us and marched down the hallway to meet the camera crew, it was exhilarating.

"Barry, I can't believe it!" I shouted. "You're going to be on national TV!"

"Don't remind me," he said. "I'm scared! I'll make a fool of myself!"

"No you won't! I'm sure you won't," I reassured him. "You have a flair for language that is better than anyone I know. You'll do fine. I'm so proud of you."

Before we got into the elevator, I gave him a big hug and kiss.

All that commotion yielded a grand total of 14 seconds of airtime for Barry. The sparse coverage was disappointing. So was the fact that the segment paid more attention to mice than human beings. The 70% reduction of Barry's cancer cited on the interview made him appear healthier than he actually was. While one tumor may have shrunk by 70%, his body was still infested with the cancer elsewhere. Yet the fact that Barry was featured on national television was a thrill, and it soon led to yet another media blitz.

On Wednesday the NBC Nightly News team tracked us down at my Aunt Helen and Uncle Joe's house in Whittier. After speeding along the LA freeways, we pulled into their driveway just one minute before the TV crew arrived. A car, a van, and a jeep were all parked in my aunt's driveway. By the time we got started it was already after 4:00 on the East Coast, and the nightly news would soon be aired.

As Barry was surrounded by a slew of lights and cameras, I could see sweat droplets streaming down his face. We handed him some cloths to wipe his brow.

"By now you're a pro at this," I said. "You'll do great!"

"I'll make a fool of myself," he said. "You just see."

"No, you won't. You'll do fine!" I said. I raced to get my own camera so I could shoot pictures of him during his interview.

"I know this sounds like an obvious question, but I'll go ahead anyway. Barry, why do you want to live?" asked the reporter over the phone.

"Because I have too many places left to visit, too many people I want to see, too many books I want to read," Barry responded. "I'd rather die in my sleep at 73 or 83 or 93, but not at 43, and not in this way."

As I glanced around the room, I could see my Uncle Joe's eyes welling up with tears. Aunt Helen was busy videotaping the filming.

In order to add some filler, the camera crew directed us for a short promenade in the backyard. Luckily all I had to do was walk beside Barry. Had I been asked to speak, I had no idea what might have come out of my mouth—I probably would have forgotten my name.

Later that evening, we all gasped when we heard Tom Brokaw's booming voice announce, "And now from Barry Riccio, in his own words...."

Before the news clip was aired, I rushed to make several phone calls. I reached my sister and asked her to phone our parents. I caught my Aunt Helen in Florida and asked her to phone our East Coast relatives. I left a message for my cousin Jack in Maine. And I repeated Monday's ritual: just before we left for the interview, I dashed off a message on the computer to our "FOB's." Over the next few days we heard from scores of friends and relatives who saw us on TV.

5/4/98 e-mail from Paul Speigel, San Francisco, CA:
Well, Kathy, that's wonderful news! Jennings couldn't have

found a better poster boy than Barry: handsome, articulate, brave and bright as hell. And my guess is that the public attention will keep the drug company from ever dropping him from the protocol.

Congratulations!
All the best to both of you!
Paul

5/4/98 e-mail from Vernon Burton and his wife Georganne, Urbana, IL:

Kathy, I also hope that this is the answer to our prayers that Barry will be cured. We miss you guys.

Love, Vernon and Georganne

5/5/98 e-mail from Mark Leff, Urbana, IL:

Kathy,

I didn't check my e-mail in time, but Georg Burton called—a few seconds too late to let me get Barry on tape, but in time to see a few seconds of his interview. Given the quality of his performance, I expect to see more of him, and I hope you'll send out future announcements.

Please tell Barry he's going to be the new Norm Ornstein.
—Mark

5/6/98 e-mail from Wendy Schmidt, Los Altos, CA:

Dear Kathy and Barry:

Alison and I watched you on NBC News tonight! I hate what they do in the media, how they reduce complexity to sound bites—'Barry Riccio the Cancer Patient.' What about Barry Riccio, the History Professor, author and playwright who has survived liver cancer for so many years with such... an experimental treatment? What about a word from his unidentified 'wife,' also a professor and author, who has much to tell the world about the advocacy role of the cancer patient's significant other in his survival? I hope you two do more press...to tell people, who suffer so widely from ignorance and fear of cancer, about the life you have been leading for the last four or five years. They need to hear more than about someone experiencing an experimental treatment that is so-far-so-good. That sounds the same as a story about AIDS research. You have both contributed so much to the experience you and others are having today in terms of your devotion to research and treatment, your zeal to know as much or more than the doctors themselves. You further the cause of a cure as much as anyone alive! It must be so gratifying to see the story of real hope begin to emerge.

Thursday we spent three hours posing for photos for *Time* Magazine. A Pulitzer-prize winning photographer and his assistant shot hundreds of pictures of us on the beach in Laguna. They asked us both to take off our shoes and socks and go barefoot.

" I don't mind going barefoot," I laughed. "But you're looking at someone else who hasn't worn sandals since he was six years old. Barry has a complex about showing his feet!"

But off came Barry's footwear, exposing all 10 pale toes. We walked along the shoreline as the photographers clicked away. Then we posed at a weather-beaten green stairway, facing some bright silver umbrellas. Later we returned to my friend's house, which was soon transformed into a studio. There Barry was asked to pose for some pensive shots.

Days later when the May 18 issue of *Time* was released, we raced to the magazine stand, frantically searching through the pages of Christine Gorman's article, "The Hope & the Hype." Ultimately the photos of us were never published, but I wrote to the editors and asked for copies, which were mailed to us in a few weeks. And although the article mentioned Barry only briefly, along with Barry's appearances on ABC and NBC, it was enough to catch the attention of a dozen or so leiomyosarcoma patients who contacted us in the upcoming months. For some time, in fact, Barry dispensed advice to desperate patients across the country.

By the time Friday was over, Barry had spent hours on the phone with journalists from *Time, The Chicago Tribune, North County Times, The Chronicle of Higher Education,* Cox News Service, and even our hometown newspaper, the Champaign-Urbana *News-Gazette.* Interspersed with this media blitz by day was a series of evening visits to family and friends in the LA area.

Things were going so well that spring I escaped on a three-week trip with my parents to Greece to visit our many relatives. I couldn't have afforded it had Mom and Dad not offered to pay for all my travel expenses. It had been six years since I had last been to Greece. After spending two summers there in the early 1990's, Barry and I had longed to return some day. But his cancer changed all that. Every year we talked about going but decided against it. Much of the medical care there—especially out on the islands—is questionable, and we didn't want to put his health in jeopardy.

Much to my surprise, during my visit I learned that several of my aunts, uncles, and cousins in Greece had seen us on television. I hadn't realized that snippets of our national news were rebroadcast on CNN International and on the Greek news. Meanwhile Barry and I spent hours faxing messages back and forth between Island Inn and Hotel Astor in Athens. I had to double-check Barry's head size so that I could stock up on some new Greek fisherman's caps.

Although I hesitated to leave Barry, I was relieved that his mother had flown out from Arizona to keep him company. Deep down I was afraid that something terrible would happen to him, and I would have to cut my trip short. But fortunately, disaster never struck. One of the highlights of the trip was when Mom and I traveled to Santorini. There we both hiked along the cliffs and drank in the spectacular scenery.

In retrospect, the trip to Greece was an excellent idea. I had missed my extended family there and was anxious to see them again. I saw several in Athens and on the island of Skyros, where we stayed for a few days. When we arrived from the Athens airport, one of my favorite relatives, Uncle George, age 87, was waiting for us in our hotel lobby. He was sitting on a couch holding his cane, surrounded by a crowd of European visitors and their usual cloud of cigarette smoke. Just a few years ago Barry and I had stayed at his modest home in Neon Hraklion and Skyros for several weeks. His house outside Athens was one of the only remaining single-family homes amidst a sea of modern high-rises. Uncle George had served as our guide to Greece and escorted us almost everywhere we went. My parents and I spent a good deal of time with him on this trip, too. During our last Sunday in Greece he joined about

20 relatives for a family reunion that Dad had organized at Erato, a charming restaurant in Plaka, the historic district of Athens. Just days after we returned to the US, Uncle George had a stroke. Sadly, only months later, he died.

Soon after Felicia left for Arizona, I returned to San Diego. At the end of June, we were invited to attend the Board of Trustees meeting at the Sidney Kimmel Cancer Center in La Jolla. At the meeting we met the three founders of the organization, Drs. Allan H. Goodman, Thomas A. Shiftan, and Ivor Royston. They spoke about the organization's progress in providing novel, non-toxic treatments for cancer patients. During their presentations they mentioned Barry and three other "success stories." All four patients were asked to stand and be acknowledged. The audience applauded enthusiastically, and I raised my hand.

"It is an honor for us to be here today," I said. "And I would like to publicly thank all of you for your efforts in saving my husband's life. We would not be here if you were not here. We are eternally grateful. And the amount of progress your organization has made in nine short years is incredible!"

As Barry put it later,

> I felt good. I was very interested to learn about SKCC. Naturally I was gratified to be "Exhibit A" in some of the talks. Listening to the speakers made me even more impatient with the romantic neo-primitivists who have long bashed science and its practical applications.

That month Barry and I belatedly celebrated our 18th wedding anniversary at Liaison, a French restaurant north of downtown. It offered an award-winning five-course dinner for two for $46, including a bottle of wine. While devouring the delectable meal, we realized that this was one of our longest stretches without bad news. Since January Barry had been receiving his weekly infusions of Vitaxin, and everything was going swimmingly. Six months was about a record for us.

We were living in a gorgeous city where the weather was perfect nearly every day. We were cool and comfortable while the rest of the country was basking in a heat wave. We relished our colorful neighborhood with its proximity to the bay and the historic Gaslamp Quarter. We enjoyed our daily waterfront walks. We treated ourselves to something special every day. We had time off from our jobs to write our books. We cherished our many visitors who came to see us from far and wide. We were spending quality time with family and friends, and most importantly, with each other. And living together in one room, we could hardly complain that we didn't see each other enough.

We missed our home, our friends, and our life in the Midwest. We missed our jobs, our colleagues, and our students. And although living in our tiny studio apartment was a hardship at times, by now all the material possessions we had left behind no longer seemed to matter. In the meantime, we had discovered something else.

Ironically, it dawned on us that the Vitaxin had offered us more than just a good quality of life. Were it not in the picture, I would have been toiling away at my job. No doubt Barry's health would have declined steadily, and chances were he would not even be alive. In fact, our quality of life was not just good. In many ways, it was even better than it would have been otherwise. It almost seemed too good to be true. And it was.

CHAPTER SEVEN

The Bubble Bursts
(1998)

"LEARNING MITIGATES THE FEAR OF DEATH."
—FRANCIS BACON

On June 30, 1998 we had arranged to meet two friends for dinner at the Vegetarian Zone. Minutes into his meal, Barry's head and neck were drenched in sweat, and his face turned yellow. He had only taken a few spoonfuls of his soup when he suddenly began vomiting over the side of the table. Our young waitress caught wind of the disaster and ran to fetch a pail and a wet washcloth. I held onto the pail in one hand and the washcloth in the other while Barry kept vomiting, one wave after another.

"Do you want to go home?" I asked him. "We can leave right now if you like. Maybe you need to get to bed."

"No, I'll be alright," he said.

I realized that our lucky spell of the past six months was now broken.

The next morning Barry felt weak and tired, so I called to schedule an emergency appointment with Dr. Kogler. After Barry explained his symptoms, Dr. Kogler asked him to go down the hall to the oncology lab for a blood test. After Barry left, the doctor reappeared.

"I purposely sent Barry to have his blood drawing now. This gives us a good opportunity to talk alone. Have you seen his latest CT-scan?" Dr. Kogler asked.

"No, I haven't," I answered.

"Unfortunately it shows a major change," he explained. "The disease is progressing, and now he is starting to show symptoms. I would consider this a treatment failure. I don't like to lie to my patients. What would you like me to say to him? I want whatever is best for him."

"Tell him the truth," I said. "And show us both the evidence. Show us this CT-scan, and let's see the other recent scans as well. I know Barry would like to know the truth. He'll also be concerned about the study. The Vitaxin was working so well for so long, and now this! Will this mean he will be kicked out of the protocol?"

"Let's leave it to Dr. Gutheil to call the shots on that. I am simply the technician here," Dr. Kogler said.

Soon after that he left the office. I stared at the four walls of the examination room, and all was eerily quiet. I was stunned by the news and on the verge of exploding into tears, but I knew that in only a few minutes both Barry and the doctor would return. I pressed my finger against my upper lip. Somewhere I had read that that could prevent one from crying. I began writing notes about what the doctor had just said. I whipped out my Stress Relief cream and dabbed more than usual on my temples, neck, and wrists. When Barry reappeared I offered him some cream. He put a small amount on his temples. Within minutes Dr. Kogler walked in.

"This time I don't need to feel you to sense your illness," said the doctor. "The CT-scan shows it, and you show it too. Here's a copy of the printout. Your cancer has grown. What concerns me especially is that the scan shows what is either fluid or cancer around the lining of the heart. Let's schedule you for an ultrasound of the heart. Also your hemoglobin is only 6.4, so you need a blood transfusion today."

The nurses in the clinic did a "type and cross" procedure for Barry's blood, and we had to wait several hours for the blood to arrive. Normally we would have gone out for a walk, but Barry was so weak that we decided to remain in the clinic. Once the packets of blood appeared he received two units. Mo, the nurse who administered Barry's transfusion, and Lisa, the nursing aid who checked his vital signs every 15 minutes, stayed long after most other staff had left for the day. The clinic normally closes at 4:30. By the time we left at 7 p.m., we had been there for over nine hours. On the way home, we made a detour for a brief walk along the waterfront at Seaport Village. After all that had happened, we both needed a breath of fresh air. Hopefully the worst was now behind us.

But at 7 a.m. the next morning, I awoke to a terrible noise. Barry was next to me, vomiting over the side of the bed. Luckily we had placed a bag there just in case. His abdomen felt bloated and tight, and his stomach was rumbling. He also had some severe lower back pain. He wanted to take a shower, but he felt so weak while washing up at the sink that I advised against it.

"Go back to bed and rest," I said. "I'll call the doctor."

By now Dr. Kogler had left for vacation, so we reached his replacement, Dr. Shiftan, who works both at Sharp Clinic and Sidney Kimmel Cancer Center. We had just seen him a few days ago at the SKCC Board meeting. He suggested that we come back to the clinic that morning. We arrived there by 10:30 and the waiting room was packed. Only one chair was free, so Barry took it. I perched myself on a small magazine stand next to him. He still looked so pale and weak that I notified Mo and Lisa behind the reception desk. They gave me a pink pail which I placed on Barry's lap just in case. After waiting for several minutes, I noticed that Barry was sweating profusely, and he was dehydrated. It appeared to be a repeat performance of the episode at Vegetarian Zone.

"I think Barry's about to faint or throw up!" I said to Mo. "Can someone come out to help us right away?"

A nurse, Diane, rushed into the waiting room and escorted Barry into the lab, where she placed him on a reclining chair. Fely, the phlebotomist, came to Barry's side and drew his blood. Every other time, Barry went to her office for this procedure, but this time she came to him. He continued to sweat non-stop. His blood test revealed that his hemoglobin was only 6.0, despite the two transfusions he had had just yesterday. The blood seemed to have gone right through him. By now we were at a loss about what to do. Soon Dr. Shiftan appeared.

"I think Barry needs to see his gastroenterologist, Dr. Pressman," he said.

"But Dr. Pressman's office is over in Hillcrest, and I don't think Barry's well enough to get over there. I don't feel comfortable driving him anywhere in this condition," I said. "I think the only place he is safe right now is either here or in the hospital."

A few minutes later Diane informed us that Dr. Shiftan arranged for Barry to be admitted to Sharp Hospital. He already had a bed assigned to him on the oncology unit on 8 North. In the meantime, Barry was still drenched in sweat, and his hair was completely soaked.

Mo asked, "Barry, do you need a wheelchair?"

"No, I'll probably be o.k.," he said.

"Good luck, Barry! Take care!" she and the other nurses called out as we left the waiting room.

By now Barry and I had come to see Mo, Lisa, Fely, Diane, and all the other nurses as friends. After all, he had seen them several times a week for almost a year and a half, and I nearly as often. They had all taken such excellent care of him, they joked around with him, and he with them. We both had grown to admire them all. I wondered whether or not Barry would be well enough to return to the clinic. Would we see all these nurses again? Or would this be a one-way trip to the hospital?

Barry leaned on me as we turned the corner into the hallway and stepped into the elevator. But before I could press the button, I could see that he was wobbly and struggling to catch his breath. He started to squat on the floor to prevent himself from falling, and I struggled to hold him up.

"Let's go get the wheelchair," I said.

At the hospital across the street, a volunteer escorted Barry upstairs. When I found him in room #858 with his nurse, Sheila, he looked like a ghost.

"Why don't you put on the hospital gown?" I suggested. "It looks like you may be here for a while."

But by now he was too weak even to think about changing his clothes.

"I'll put it on later," he said. "I don't feel like it right now."

Within seconds Barry began to vomit with a vengeance. Watching him throw up so violently three times in one day—and black blood at that—was a shock to me. I didn't think a human being could survive this kind of episode, and I couldn't help but fear that the end was near. How did Barry feel?

> Awful! It was probably the most uncomfortable day of my life. I didn't have the luxury of being philosophical. I was focusing on making the next step…staying conscious and not vomiting more than was necessary.

Later that evening Dr. Shiftan appeared.

"Do you have Power of Attorney?" he asked. "You'll have to think about whether or not you want to continue treatment if the situation can not be turned around."

I could feel my heart racing as I digested the doctor's words.

"I don't want to remain a vegetable," Barry said.

In fact, we had already filled out the forms.

Later that evening, Dr. Pressman, the gastroenterologist, appeared for Barry's endoscopy. Before giving Barry the anesthesia the doctor asked Barry to describe the Haymarket Riots in Chicago. But after only a few sentences, Barry was knocked out. Eventually the test revealed that the tumor in his stomach muscle lining was extensive, but it was obscured by a massive amount of blood.

By now Barry had become philosophical about the past few days. "'Yesterday' was not just a Beatles song to me. It was more like Dante's Ninth Circle of Hell."

During the next few days a number of doctors paraded through Barry's room. Even a social worker came to discuss matters with us. First Dr. Shiftan appeared; then a surgeon, Dr. Barone; and then another gastroenterologist, Dr. Snyder, substituting for Dr. Pressman.

Dr. Barone said to us, "I am one of the most aggressive surgeons west of the Mississippi. I am more than willing to operate. But I should tell you that it would be a complicated, messy procedure. I might get in there and have to take out your colon. I might have to remove your entire stomach and put you on feeding tubes for the rest of your life. I could also strike a major blood vessel and cause significant bleeding. In fact several patients have died when I have tried this kind of procedure on them."

Barry considered the doctor's comments.

Later he said to me, "I am a risk taker but within reasonable limits. And this sounds unreasonable. I am beginning to think this is a one-way trip on the Titanic."

When Dr. Snyder arrived, he took one look at Barry and said, "Jeffrey (Pressman, the gastroenterologist) thinks you're a phenomenon."

Since he could see Barry was uncomfortable with the nasogastric tube, he removed it. After having been at the hospital almost six hours that day, I left around 7:00 p.m., absolutely exhausted. I drove to La Jolla, where I had dinner with my parents. That night after taking a Tylenol PM, I slept well for the first time in several days.

Bright and early on the 4th of July, Barry had a chest x-ray. Dr. Barone and Dr. Shiftan stopped by to visit, and then he went for a mile-long walk around the oncology ward. The doctors told him about a drug called Procrit that boosts the hemoglobin level. He would need to start taking it as soon as possible.

By the time I arrived at the hospital early that afternoon, I heard the patient two doors away from Barry's room howling away.

He was screaming, "I'm so hungry! I'm so hungry! No more ice chips!" and "Let me out of here! Let me out of here!"

It sounded more like an insane asylum than a cancer ward. We found out that his name was Randy, and that he had been in that hospital room for over a month.

According to Barry, he was "both comical and haunting at the same time."

Although I felt sorry for Randy, his shrieks became increasingly grating. It turns out that the only time he stopped howling was when he was drugged up, asleep, or when his mother came to visit.

Later that day Barry had an MRI, a test he had only had twice before. Since his condition was so complex, the MRI needed to examine the chest, abdomen, and pelvis, and the test would take longer than usual. He was given a white washcloth to place over his eyes, and two yellow earplugs. Here is how Barry described his procedure.

> I felt like a prisoner. I felt trapped. The clanging noises
> were reminiscent of what one might hear in a torture session at
> a concentration camp. I became very, very hot. I was pro-

foundly uncomfortable because I'm not accustomed to lying on my back for that long a period of time. And I knew when I was halfway done that I couldn't do it all in one day.

I was trying to think of books I had read and places I had gone, but I couldn't really think too much as I was in far too much pain. Near the end I thought surely there was a simpler way to get this information. It makes the CT-scan seem like a picnic.

When I came out I said, "That must have been about 40 minutes, wasn't it?"

But it was only about 20. I could write a book about torture now... Medical Torture, American Style...For the upper GI test I was turning in all directions. For the bone scan I was strapped down like a mummy. And now this....

I accompanied Barry for the MRI. Before entering the room, I had to leave my purse, wallet, calculator, and laptop computer in a locker. If not, the machine could wipe out everything on the magnetic strips. I was seated in a white wicker rocking chair across the room from Barry. The machine was mammoth.

"I hope I never have to have one of these," I thought to myself.

All I could see was a bit of Barry's black hair and his hands cupped together over his head. I saw his wedding ring, a sheet, a pillow, and a pad below. I heard a set of tapping sounds, almost like at a construction site. Now another set of tapping sounds, first like bongo drums, then a construction drill. Then the drill again several times. At times it sounded like a machine gun. The lights above the machine showed numbers marked "Scanning...#....Remaining." The numbers kept running from 406 to 0, and then the process was repeated all over again. During Barry's tests I was taking notes, and I stopped for a moment to study my pen. It was from the Borrego Springs Resort Hotel, which we had visited just a few months ago. We had hiked up a canyon to see the spring wildflowers. Although we had only been there in April, it seemed like years ago.

"What a way to spend the Fourth of July," I thought. "Just think of all the picnics and parties going on all over the country. And here we are, back in the hospital. But I suppose it's better than being stuck in the hospital at Christmas time. We've been through that twice before."

When Barry finally escaped from the machine, he was drenched. The technicians told him to remain there for another several minutes, and they informed me that my parents were waiting upstairs.

Barry postponed the rest of the test until the next day. He couldn't take any more of that torture chamber. So my parents, the transporter, and I wheeled him back up to his room, where he awaited an additional blood transfusion. I left at about 6:00. Even though it had only been five hours, it felt like a very long day. Although I was exhausted, I didn't want the holiday to pass me by. I drove to La Jolla where I joined Mom and Dad for dinner. Then we took a short drive to La Jolla Cove. Kellogg Park was crammed with picnickers and other spectators who must have staked out their spots hours ago. Without an inch to spare on the grass, we carved out a spot for three and leaned on some parked cars. From there, with palm trees silhouetted in the foreground, we viewed a spectacular fireworks display straight overhead. Never before had I seen them so close. Add to that live music, and it was the best 4th of July celebration I had ever seen. And for a few moments, I forgot about all the vomiting, the blood transfusions, and the claustrophobic MRI.

After spending the night at my parents' house, the next morning I dashed over to the hospital just in time to catch Dr. Shiftan. He discussed, among other things, the merits of radiation to try to stop Barry's bleeding.

"If Barry is taken off the Vitaxin, and we decide to go back home to Illinois, do you think he is well enough to make the cross-country drive?" I asked.

The doctor raised his eyebrows and replied, "As we've seen this past week, his situation could turn around very quickly. I certainly wouldn't do it if I were you! Leave the car here."

Was the famous study now over? And the miracle drug a failure? Would we be heading back home soon? Would I be going back to work that fall? All these questions were spinning around my head that day. Later that morning we met with Dr. Barone.

"I've reviewed the results of all Barry's tests in the meantime," he told us, "and now I would strongly advise against surgery. The risks are simply too great. Radiation is the best route at this point."

Fortunately, this was the first day that Barry looked and sounded more like his normal self. His hemoglobin had stabilized in the 9 range, and the night before, while I was watching fireworks at the Cove, he had walked a mile in the hospital. We walked another mile together around the oncology ward, around and around in circles. Then I took him upstairs to the hospital's rooftop deck to get some fresh air.

The following day Barry completed his MRI. This time he was given stronger relaxing medication. He was also able to listen to some music, and that helped. Since he was so exhausted from lack of sleep, he rested during the test, which was less grueling than before. He also had an ultrasound of the heart. At 6 p.m. Dr. Kogler arrived and we chatted for about 45 minutes. He had just returned from his 4th of July weekend. I asked Dr. Kogler the same questions I had asked Dr. Shiftan.

"You have to realize that now the situation has changed. *You are sitting on a barrel of dynamite!* Barry could bleed at any time. Let's try to prevent a repeat performance of last week. Bring Barry in to the clinic every morning to have his hemoglobin level checked. And on the weekends when the clinic is closed, have him checked at the hospital. I will place a standing order for the blood tests. At the first sign of trouble, we could try to get the situation under better control."

Later that evening Dr. Scott arrived. He had been Barry's radiation oncologist for his head tumor last fall.

"Radiation on your stomach will make you as sick as a dog!" he told us. "It's a miserable process. Right now it would be a shotgun approach. Let's wait in case your bleeding stops on its own. Then there's no point putting you through it now. It might jeopardize your staying on in the protocol, although I hope not. If you continue bleeding and we just can't seem to stop it any other way, then let's radiate right away. I might be able to stop the bleeding in just a few hours."

The next day Dr. Barone stopped by to check on Barry.

"The MRI showed the upper right quadrant of the abdomen is all tumor. Now I definitely think that surgery just won't work."

Not only was the stomach all socked with tumor; now so was much of the abdomen. With that news, we walked around in circles in 8 North, a total of two miles. Since there was little else that could be done at this point besides administering blood transfusions, it was time for

Barry to be released. Nonetheless, we had to wait for Dr. Pressman to give the official dismissal. We waited all day for him, and he finally appeared at 7:15 that evening.

"I think so much of you two," he told us. "I'm so sorry that you both have to go through this. Barry, you've fought a good fight. But you can't win every battle. Even the best Generals lose the war! Look at Robert E. Lee. He was one of the world's best Generals, but he couldn't win the Civil War.

"After a certain point you'll just have to agree that it was a heroic fight, but now I lost the battle, and that's o.k. Yet I still see a fighting spirit, and now is probably not that time. You'll know when that is. You'll know. You know, I probably shouldn't tell you this, but when I first met you last summer, I thought you'd be dead in 12 weeks. If I were in your shoes I would have been dead long ago. You've done better than anyone."

"So what should we do now?" we asked.

"Barry, your stomach tumor is pressing on your small intestine, and the opening from the stomach is very, very small. You just can't eat like you used to. You need to stay on full liquids only. This means yogurts, puddings, custards, pureed foods, mashed potatoes, applesauce, ice cream, frozen yogurts, baby foods, cream soups, scrambled eggs."

"How about cream of wheat?" Barry asked.

"O.k."

"How about oatmeal?"

"No. No chunks of anything. You need to be able to pour the food...it's got to be really soft. Do you have a blender?"

"Not here," I replied. "We have one in Urbana, but not in San Diego."

"Go out and buy one right away," said the doctor. "You can't get by without it. And be sure to eat frequent but small meals. And don't eat any less than two hours before sleeping. You want to be sure not to block the opening of the stomach."

"In the future, how do we know what's an emergency and what's not? How do we prevent a scenario like last week's from happening again?" I asked.

"If he throws up blood—either fresh red blood or old brown blood—or he throws up food many times, he needs to be in the hospital. If he throws up just a little food, then he's o.k. at home. Keep a close eye on him.

"My advice to you now is to enjoy each other and the days you have together. Spend quality time with each other. Go out and watch the sun set over the ocean every night. Why not catch it tonight? There's going to be a good one.

"And laugh. Laugh as much as you can. Here are some videos you might want to rent. Do you have a VCR?"

"Not here," I said. "We have one in Urbana, but not here."

"I can lend you an extra one from my house if you like. Just let me know," said Dr. Pressman.

With that he pulled out his prescription pad and jotted down his favorite comedies.

"Good luck to both of you," he said.

And then he left. Although I half expected this conversation, it still came as a shock. How did Barry feel?

> I was taken aback. It was not unlike the reaction I had when I first was told that I had cancer five years earlier. It almost seemed unbelievable at first. Since January and February, when I was doing so well on the Vitaxin study, I stopped referring to myself as *terminal.* I really thought that I had five to 10 years left. But somehow now I feel even worse about the food. I'm not going to prance around eating Gerber's at this stage! At least I always liked pureed soups and ice cream.

"Well, let's just take the doctor's advice," I said to Barry. "Take a look at this scene out the window."

And with that we watched a spectacular sunset over Mount Soledad. The sky turned bright pink behind a parade of cumulus clouds.

At 8:30 that evening Barry checked out of the hospital and we headed back to Island Inn. Although his stay there had only been five days, it felt as if it had been all summer long. The next morning while Barry was still sleeping, I walked over to Ralph's grocery store and searched up and down the aisles for the kinds of food that Barry could eat. I stocked up on puddings, applesauce, and several flavors of yogurt, as much as could fit in our tiny refrigerator.

Later we drove across town to Target in search of a blender. It seemed as if everything we saw was now in black and white, and only the restaurants appeared in color. Coco's, Denny's, Taco Bell, Burger King...even places at which we rarely ate popped out at us like never before. In my mind, each was marked with a big red X, like a scarlet letter. Forbidden! And what was Barry thinking?

> The clouds of unreality gathered around me most of the day. The stringency of my new diet began to sink in. I felt awkward walking by a popcorn stand and smelling it, not unlike Ulysses when he was chained to the mast and hearing the songs of the sirens. He was tempted to meet with them but couldn't because of the constraints under which he was placed.
>
> We walked into a shop at Seaport Village called The Garlic Patch. I was not sorely tempted there, but I did discover to my relief a recipe for scrambled eggs in a tiny garlic recipe book.

As I watched Barry studying the jars of garlic ale mustard and garlic barbecue sauce, I recalled how many hours we used to spend in shops like these—whether it was here in California, in Chicago, in Kansas City, or in other cities we visited. We would find the most exotic items to fill our kitchen cupboards, and Barry would create some delicious concoctions with them. Now all that was behind us. I was on the verge of tears, and Barry was depressed.

> I'll never be able to have stuffed shells Sorrento again, my famous barbecued meatballs, or barbecued beef or chicken sandwiches. I had a taste for Larry Blake's barbecue sauce which is the best in the country...thick and rich in molasses and brown sugar. No more bulgogi, beef panang, pasta, gnocchi...

Barry described his latest setback in this 7/13/98 e-mail from Barry to Anita Shelton, Chair of the History Department, Eastern Illinois University, Charleston, IL; San Diego, CA

Subject: The Bubble Burst

Hi Anita,

I hope all is well with you. Have you had your marathon yet? And how did the Fourth of July birthday party for Joy go? My Fourth was spent inside a hospital. The enemy within returned two weeks ago, and with a vengeance. The details are too gruesome for me to go into over the computer, but the upshot is that my cancer has grown in my liver and stomach. Unlike the 1993 and 1995 incidents, though, this time the stomach cancer cannot be removed surgically. Too many other organs would have to be removed, and too many crucial blood vessels would be at risk. Radiation, I am told, would make me "sick as a dog" and not even eliminate the tumor. When I bleed again — and I bled like hell a week and a half ago — I will need the radiation, if only for a few days, just to stop the bleeding. The biggest change, however, involves my eating habits. I'll never be able to have "normal" food again. In fact, from now on everything I eat must have the consistency of baby food. I always was overly preoccupied with food. Now, of course, I obsess about it more than ever.

You're probably wondering why this happened, after all the publicity about my success. Well, it turns out that only about a third of my tumors were being "tracked." Those tumors actually did quite well until recently, of course. But that was only a part of the story. It appears that my body built up a resistance, on the one hand, and responded very unevenly to the antibody, on the other. Since the database for this drug is so small, and since a quarter of the "guinea pigs" have died already, the doctors don't seem especially surprised by my turn for the worse. To some extent, the shock has even worn off of me. After all, I did receive three previous death sentences. This one (which gives me about a year or so) can't be easily dismissed. There is so much more cancer in my body now, I'm beginning to feel the pain, and I'm already thirty pounds thinner than I was two summers ago, when I received the last notice. The boy who cried "Wolf" did prove to be right in the end, after all.

Fortunately, neither the doctors nor the biotech company

want me off the study as of yet. In the (admittedly unlikely) possibility that this drug is still doing a modicum of good, they are beginning the eighth round tomorrow. Ixsys certainly has nothing to lose. There are no longer any supply problems, no one else is demanding the drug at the moment (we are in between protocols), and the longer I'm kept on the drug the better it looks for the company. But I told the lead physician that when he came to the conclusion that the drug was no longer doing any good whatsoever, I would certainly not quarrel with the result.

I'm sorry to be the bearer of bad tidings, but it appears that the "miracle man" is out of miracles.

Best,

Barry

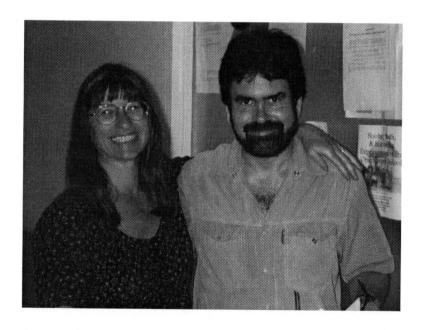

Barry and his department chair, Anita Shelton, at Eastern Illinois University. Because Barry's days were numbered, Anita led the effort to accelerate his tenure process. Charleston, Illinois; July 1996. (credit: Dan Crews)

7/15/98 e-mail from Anita Shelton to Barry
Charleston, IL:

Dear Barry,

I hate to think of you under siege or tormented in any
way. I cannot bear the idea of losing you. You are a marvelous,
idiosyncratic, lovely, funny, odd, bright, committed, sincere
and courageous person. You showed your courage long before
your illness, by the way, in the way that you lived through all
the years of (completely undeserved) professional limbo;
however frustrated or disappointed, you never seemed sour or
whiny (as so many academics do, even when they are "successful"). I marvel at your sincere love of your chosen field of study.
I like the partnership of you and Kathy as a couple (not true of
many couples), in your lovely southwestern-flavored home. I
like the way (as Casey described it) you would go to Timpone's,
analyze every item on the menu and then always order the
same pizza. I have missed so much your purple shirts and
slightly fuddled manner. I don't know what to say in response
to your last message, except to try to tell you how much I
respect and care for you, have missed you since you left, and
am so saddened that you are facing what you are facing.

Are you able to say at this point whether you expect still to
be coming out this way in August or not? Can the doctors give
you medication for pain without making you groggy? How is
Kathy holding up? Please give her my warmest regards.

I have passed your message on to others in the department, thinking that they would also want to contact you; I
hope that's all right.

Sadly, and with deep and fierce affection,

Anita

By now Barry's cancer was in his stomach, liver, abdomen wall,
spleen, belly cavity, lesser omentum, mesentery, his mediastinum, and
near the pericardium. In retrospect, it seemed that the Vitaxin had

succeeded in keeping the cancer in his liver at bay, and stalling its growth elsewhere. It had been the finger in the dike. And it held up longer than I ever would have dreamed was possible. Given that it had virtually no side effects, I still consider it a medical miracle. But eventually the monster caught up with him, and once again the bullets aimed right at us.

Much to our surprise, Dr. Gutheil and Ixsys allowed Barry to remain on the Vitaxin. Despite this recent setback, the tests did not reveal that the drug was doing him any harm. And since he was now on the compassionate use protocol, the restrictions of the Phase 1 research study no longer applied. As long as he continued on the drug we would need to remain out West. As a result, I once again put our return to Urbana on hold. Unlike last year, now Barry's condition was so serious that I couldn't even consider leaving him alone. My colleagues were more than accommodating. I spoke with one of them by phone.

"Take your time and do what you need to do," she advised. "I have discussed your situation with our director, and you can return whenever you like. Don't worry."

I realized how lucky I was to have a job like mine, because anywhere else after so many months of uncertainty, I might have been fired. After speaking with my colleague, the pressure to return to work subsided.

In the meantime, Barry managed to survive on the pureed diet, although it was not easy. Our tiny quarters at Island Inn prevented us from doing much cooking. We still ate out about once a day, but now we often called in advance to see if the chefs could prepare a pureed soup, mashed potatoes, or scrambled eggs. Most staff went out of their way to serve us. I made special trips to the deli bar at Whole Foods grocery store, where I bought delicious chili and other pureed soups for Barry. These were special treats. When we were on the go, we carried an insulated thermos bag full of applesauce and small snacks. I bought several containers of Ensure, a nutritional supplement, to keep Barry's weight up. Nonetheless, he still looked gaunt, especially after his recent hospital stay.

How did Barry deal with all his dietary constraints?

> I'm not all that worried about the cancer in my liver and my abdomen except for what's in my stomach. I worry about that more because of the future. I wonder at what point I'll be told I can't eat anything. I sense the ticking time bomb more in my stomach than in any other part of my body.
>
> I'm handling the diet well but I'm still frustrated from time to time about not being able to eat certain types of food. I'm more than willing to be on this diet if I have to be, but I would like to have the right to cheat at least once a week.

While he obeyed Dr. Pressman's advice for another month or two, finally he caved in.

One day he called the doctor and asked, "May I try going off this diet one day a week?"

"Go ahead and try it and see what happens," the doctor advised. "But be careful."

His first real meal was at The Old Spaghetti Factory, where he ordered spaghetti and meatballs. It was a restaurant near us in the Gaslamp Quarter where we had eaten many times with my family, a place with sentimental value to both of us. I flashed back to our first meal there together almost 20 years ago. It was after a long summer day at the beach and Barry had came down with a ferocious sunburn. The first time I ever touched him was that day, to apply Solarcaine all over his back and arms. During dinner his feet had been so swollen that he had to remove his shoes, something he rarely did in public.

I was mulling over this scene as the host seated us in an old trolley car with a panoramic view of the dining room. As always I had hidden the pink pail in my bag just in case Barry couldn't make it to the restroom on time. I was on edge as he began swallowing his pasta and chewing his garlic bread.

"Take your time, Barry! Eat slowly! And remember, you don't have to finish your meal. You can take some of it home with you!" I said to him.

Much to my chagrin, he proceeded to devour his spaghetti with record speed.

"What if something goes wrong, and he vomits in full view of the whole restaurant?" I thought to myself. "This is a disaster waiting to happen."

But nothing did. Encouraged by the success of his first experiment, Barry gradually found more occasions to test his ability to digest normal food. In late August, while at Seaport Village with a friend, he ate a Chicago-style pizza topped with pineapple and jalapeño peppers.

"Why did you have to have two pieces of that pizza?" I chided him. "That's only common sense. That pizza is sitting like a brick in your stomach."

"But I only had two pieces," he said. "Usually I would have four."

Although it never tasted better to him, it came out with a vengeance. His hemoglobin dropped and he was administered blood transfusions the next day. Later that week he had a craving for a keema curry dish with rice at World Curry, one of our favorite eateries in Pacific Beach. Bruce, the owner, even pureed it for him, but at Barry's insistence, he made it spicy.

"Why can't you have it mild, just to be on the safe side?" I asked.

"Because I always have it spicy," he replied.

Later that evening he felt that brick back in his stomach again, and no matter if he stood, sat, or laid down, he couldn't get comfortable. He threw up twice overnight and ended up in the Emergency Room at 6:30 the next morning. He was back in the hospital on 8 North for another several days. From then on it seemed as if almost any time he bent the rules, he began vomiting dark brown blood. I tried to be his food police, but to no avail.

By early September I counted up some statistics. Since he was first diagnosed with cancer he had received nearly 50 blood transfusions. He had spent 62 days of his life in the hospital. His sagging trousers reminded him that he must have been losing weight, but when the scale showed him to be a meager 156 pounds, he was shocked.

"For the first time I began to wonder if I only had weeks left rather than a year or two—just a fleeting thought that crossed my mind," he said.

In the meantime, we visited Sharp Infusion Therapy Center every weekday. Dr. Kogler had ordered that Barry receive a transfusion whenever his hemoglobin fell below 7. From July on he needed transfusions anywhere from one to three times a week. Usually he could wait for a transfusion the next day, but sometimes his hemoglobin level dropped so quickly that he needed a transfusion that same day. Soon he became a permanent fixture at the clinic, so much so that he even gravitated regularly to a favorite chair, the third one in the second row. After a while it almost had his name on it. Barry kept himself busy by reading books and newspapers that he brought in from home and by chatting with other patients. Just as he had been "King of International House" as a student, he was now "King of the Clinic" as a patient. Most of the patients knew him by name and enjoyed talking with him.

By now the transfusion procedure had become routine. At the clinic Fely, the phlebotomist, drew Barry's blood. She had a playful spirit and a musical voice.

"Barry, your turn," she would say as she called him from the waiting room.

After taking her sample, she would bandage up Barry's arm in a color to match whatever shirt he was wearing. Whether it was a red, teal, blue, or purple shirt, she always had a bandage to match.

Mo almost always administered Barry's transfusions and Lisa checked his vital signs.

Whenever Lisa saw him walk in the door to the waiting room, she would bow to greet him, "Hello, Your Highness!"

And he would respond, "Hello, My Liege!"

His other nurses included Joan, Diane, June, and Cindy. All the nurses were top notch, caring and compassionate without being patronizing to their patients. I especially admired Mo, who went out of her way to create an upbeat environment in what could have been a depressing place. She decorated the clinic with red, white, and blue streamers for the Fourth of July; purple and green palm tree streamers for summer; and San Diego Padres memorabilia for fall. When the team made it to the World Series, she even set up a tailgate party in the clinic complete with onion dip, tortilla chips, cucumbers, carrots, celery, and Halloween cookies. Oddly enough, the ambience at the clinic almost made us want to come to the doctor's office. It was a pleasant sensation!

On weekends we made daily visits to Sharp Hospital, where the staff was equally friendly but the process much slower. Most of the time Barry was transfused with two units. As a result, whenever he needed a transfusion in the hospital, it usually turned out to be an all-day affair. Sometimes the transfusions lasted until 11:00 p.m. On rare occasions he began the process in the evening, stayed overnight in the hospital, and was released early the next morning.

Often I waited with him for a good part of the day or at least until the blood arrived, and sometimes I stayed with Barry throughout the nine-hour ordeal. But other times I grew impatient, accompanying him to his hospital room and then returning later that day. It was hard for me to sit still for that long. And I had spent so many hours in hospitals that I relished the times I could get away from them. Whenever possible I escaped to my parents' house in La Jolla where I often squeezed in a quick swim. That refreshment kept me going for the rest of the day. Barry's mother, however, could sit still longer than I could. Whenever she visited she kept him company throughout the transfusion process, whether it was in the hospital or in the clinic.

"What do you think of your daily trips to the clinic?" I asked him.

> It's like my job. I'd rather be monitored too much than too little, given my situation. Given that that's what I'm out here to do, I can't quarrel with that. That's my primary purpose for being here. I think very highly of the people who are treating me.
>
> I also feel better that I don't have to fight to get the Vitaxin any more. Dr. Gutheil suggested that I can either have the radiation on my stomach apart from the Vitaxin, as I did last year when my head was radiated. Or I can have it simultaneously with the radiation this time.

"And how about food? What are your thoughts on that these days?" I asked.

> I'm afraid of food these days. Clearly my gastronomic satisfactions are not what they used to be. I understand that. It's awkward not to be able to eat what I want. So I have to look forward to other things. I've turned to my books, I've turned to my plays, I've turned to my films. For the longest time I've derived much of my satisfaction from walking. Lately I can't do that much either, but I trust that will change soon.

That fall Dr. Scott began administering the radiation he had discussed with us earlier in the summer. Barry went to his office for radiation five times a week for six weeks, split into two segments: four weeks on radiation, six weeks on Vitaxin, followed by two more weeks on radiation. Ironically, since Barry had already been sick as a dog, the treatment didn't make him feel any worse.

We were never certain how effective the radiation was. On the one hand, Dr. Scott's assistants seemed to believe that it was working. But on the other hand, as the fall continued, Barry got sicker and sicker. Clearly there was more cancer in his body than there had been before.

———————

October ended with a bang. Barry spent most of Halloween in the hospital after a bout of non-stop vomiting. He started in the morning with a few hours of respite in the hospital, where his nurse informed him that his lab tests indicated there was no need for a blood transfusion that day. Immediately after returning home, he began vomiting once again. Two friends were visiting from the Bay Area. Since Barry was feeling under the weather, I joined them for a late lunch. Later that evening Barry vomited yet again. Within an hour of his last vomiting episode Barry felt well enough to go for a walk and observe the unusual costumes parading around the Gaslamp Quarter. The next day Barry recovered. He was even able to eat a baked potato for dinner. Although he was still obsessed about "vomiting my guts out," nothing happened. After our friends left Barry began to eat more normal food, a little each day at a time. By the middle of November he was eating just about all he wanted. Since we were to celebrate his birthday away from home one more time, and since I was never certain just how many more birthdays Barry would reach, I sent out a secret note to our support group.

11/14/98 e-mail from me to Friends of Barry
San Diego, CA:

> To our FOB's (Friends of Barry): Just a quick note to let you know that Barry's 44th birthday is Sunday, November 15. There have been many days when I thought he'd never get there, so it is definitely time to celebrate.

So how about an e-mail surprise party? If you like, you can send birthday greetings to him directly at cfbdr@eiu.edu.

I'll send an update on his health situation in the next month or so along with our e-mail holiday newsletter. It's a long story, but as of today, he is doing well. He just completed round #9 of the Vitaxin study and is undergoing radiation treatments. Our good friend, Amita Sinha, from Champaign, along with his mother, has joined us here in San Diego for the festivities.

I wish you all an early Happy Thanksgiving! –Kathy

Within the next several days he heard from hundreds of people. The surprise party had been a success. In addition to celebrating at Ember's, one of our favorite restaurants, we strolled around Balboa Park and saw a suspenseful thriller on stage at the Torrey Pines Theater in La Jolla. Our friend, Amita, had flown out from Champaign to join us. All in all it was a festive day.

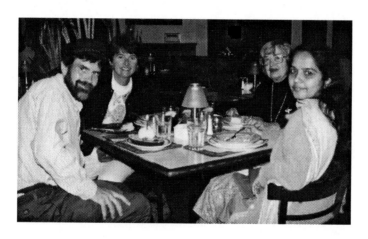

Celebrating Barry's 44th birthday with his mother, Felicia Riccio, and Amita Sinha, who visited us from Champaign. That day scores of friends from around the country contributed to his virtual surprise birthday party over electronic mail. San Diego, California; November 1998. (credit: unknown)

As the holiday season approached I felt a sense of impending doom, and I feared that another downturn was imminent. So I decided to take advantage of all the local festivities, to make hay while the sun was shining, so to speak. During the first two weeks of December it seems as if we went to almost every Christmas event listed in *The San Diego Reader*. We witnessed the lavish tree lighting ceremony at the Hotel del Coronado. We heard the Singing Christmas tree, a group of church carolers perched atop platforms in the shape of a Christmas tree, at Seaport Village. We joined thousands of revelers for Christmas on the Prado in Balboa Park. We saw the Christmas parade in downtown La Jolla. We enjoyed the historical candlelight spectacle of Las Posadas at Old Town. I have no regrets about overindulging in the holiday spirit, for in a few days our roller coaster ride would take yet another descent.

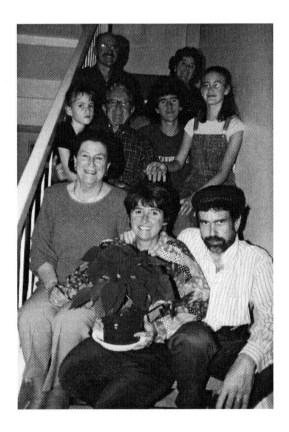

Thanksgiving with my sister's family. Due to his serious liver problems, this was the last time Barry drank a full glass of wine. L-R back row: John Smith, my brother-in-law, and Mary Anne Anthony Smith, my sister. Middle row: Jeannette Smith, Dad, Alexander Smith, Annie Smith. Front row: Mom, myself, Barry. Irvine, California: November 1998. (credit: unknown)

One afternoon during a lunch at our favorite Indian restaurant, Dan spotted a growth above Barry's upper lip, under his mustache. Barry had seen it a few days earlier but didn't know what to make of it. Both of us had hoped it was merely a pimple, as we had once thought about the growth on Barry's head. Yet deep down we both dreaded what it could mean.

"I hate to say this, but I think it could be another tumor," Dan said. "Have your doctor take a look at it."

With that my curry dish began churning in my stomach. In early December Barry met with both Dr. Scott, the radiation oncologist, and Dr. Y, the head surgeon. Without even taking a biopsy, they confirmed that the growth was cancerous.

I thought to myself, "The cancer had hit him all over his gut, then knocked him on the head, and now it even punched him in the face. What more can go wrong?"

Dr. Scott hesitated to radiate the region since it could end up closing Barry's mouth forever, making him unable to speak or eat. Dr. Y preferred surgery but he couldn't do it alone.

So he and Dr. Kogler referred us to yet another physician, a plastic surgeon who specialized in the face. We visited his office early one morning and met with him for an hour. He was very pleasant and informative. But what he said was downright chilling.

"The surgery will leave you with a large scar on your face. I'm afraid that it won't be concealed by your beard or mustache. Even though the tumor is small, we'll need to cut out a wide margin. For two and a half weeks you'll barely be able to open your mouth, and you'll have to eat everything through a tiny, narrow straw. By the way, you don't have any problem vomiting, do you?" asked the doctor.

With that my hair began to stand on end.

"Yes, he certainly does!" I replied. "I'm afraid of seeing him have an operation like that under these conditions. He's been vomiting regularly. Couldn't he end up choking on his own vomit? I know someone who died that way."

"You're right," said the doctor. "That's a risk you'd have to take."

As we descended towards the parking garage, I told Barry, "I'm not going to let you have that operation."

We had already scheduled it with the doctor, but after learning how dangerous it could be, I chickened out. Our meeting with Dr. Kogler the next day confirmed my suspicions.

"Let's wait on the lip," he said. "You're not ready for that now. Maybe we can get at it some other way. Not only is vomiting a concern, but so is your low hemoglobin. It needs to be at least 10 to withstand an operation, and yours has been much lower than that."

After leaving Dr. Kogler's office, we called the plastic surgeon to cancel the operation. It reminded me of when Barry's operation in Detroit was canceled at the last minute, only this time we had a day to spare.

In December 1998 a combination of Italian, Greek, and Mexican food led to another gut-wrenching episode. Within four days he vomited those horribly familiar coffee grounds five times. But this time he couldn't keep down any food at all, not even a spoonful of yogurt or a cup of tea. His stomach felt bloated and his abdomen hard as a rock. After a late-night trip to the Emergency Room, he was sent home.

Two days later Dr. Pressman performed an endoscopy on Barry. It had been several months since he had last had that test. When the doctor came to meet me, his face looked grim.

"I hate to tell you this, but the news is not good," said Dr. Pressman. "Barry's got a blood clot and the tumor is bleeding. He needs to be admitted to the hospital. His condition is very serious. I'm so sorry you both have to go through this. You're both too young."

When I went back into the recovery room, I saw Barry's shoes listlessly dangling over the gurney. His body was limp, his face white, and his eyes rolled over. Although he was just regaining consciousness, seeing him like that took my breath away. He looked as if he were dead. Once again I began to think that this would be a one-way trip to the hospital. After a few days in the hospital Dr. Gutheil came by his room.

"The bleeding just doesn't seem to be stopping and your cancer is growing," he said. "It's clear to me that the Vitaxin isn't working anymore. You certainly got a lot of mileage out of it—10 rounds— more than anyone expected. Yet now it might even be contributing to your bleeding. It's time to stop it. I actually think that now you're better off on chemotherapy."

His words rang like the chimes of a clock tower. There was no doubt that the study was over.

As Barry put it, "It was the end of the Vitaxin era."

And it was the moment we had been dreading for so long. But there was no point in putting up a fight, because it was obvious even to us that this time the doctors were right. His cancer was definitely getting worse—and now out of control. Ironically by now the staff at Ixsys would not have minded keeping Barry on the drug even longer, as he had become their poster boy. And there were no longer any supply problems. We agreed to stop the treatment.

Once again a parade of doctors appeared in Barry's hospital room. After a series of tests, Dr. Kogler and Dr. Pressman concluded that there were only two options now available: 1) a permanent gastric feeding tube or 2) surgery to remove the obstruction.

We met with Dr. Barone to discuss the possibility of surgery.

"Barry, he explained, "I have some patients who tell me that no matter what, they just want to eat a hamburger. They don't care if they die on the operating table. They just want to eat that hamburger! Are you one of those people? I have to ask you this, because I must tell you that this kind of bypass operation is extremely dangerous. There's a 50:50 chance of success, and a 10% chance that you could die during the surgery. We could run into enormous liver and bleeding complications. I've seen it happen many times. But it's also possible that it could work. You tell me!"

"I don't think I'm ready for that just now. I've been a risk taker in the past, but this sounds like just too big a risk to take," Barry said.

I heaved a sigh of relief. There's no way I would have gone ahead with that surgery after hearing the doctor's warning. With that, the feeding tube was our last resort. Now the man who loved to eat would no longer eat at all. To make matters worse, Dr. Pressman had told us earlier that even inserting the gastric tube could lead to complications—and possibly be fatal. Barry's condition was so complex that the doctor might not even be able to insert the tube at all. He was left with a Catch 22.

What were Barry's thoughts at the time?

> I don't like this. It doesn't seem very appealing. But now it's not about solutions. It's about survival.

A nurse came to Barry's room that evening and explained at great length exactly how the feeding tube would be inserted and how to care for it. From her perspective it was a very easy process. But to us it sounded extremely complex. The scene reminded me of the cows I used to drive by at the South Farms of our University of Illinois campus, the ones with those ugly holes that allow researchers to study their digestive systems. I spent that night at my parents' house in La Jolla, where I had camped out since Barry entered the hospital.

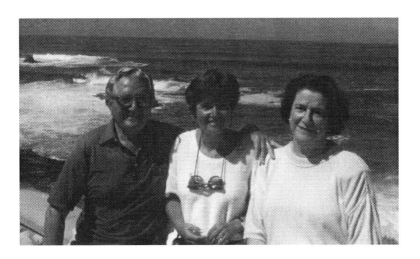

My parents, Harry and Anne Anthony, were a steady source of support for both of us during our stay in San Diego. I saw them more during the two years we spent there than I had in the previous decade. San Diego, California; July 1997. (credit: Barry Riccio)

Mom cooked a wonderful meal for me as I described the day's saga. When I got into bed I relished the familiar feel of flannel sheets, something I had missed for months.

"How lucky I am to have Mom and Dad nearby," I thought, "and especially at a time like this. If I were back home alone in Illinois, I might be falling apart."

Yet I could hardly sleep. Images of Barry, the feeding tube, and those cows kept spinning around my head. Had it finally come to this? What more could go wrong? To me we had crossed another threshold, the point of no return. The doctors had always mentioned the need for a good quality of life. Now even that would be stolen from Barry.

Our mood was morose the next morning as we sensed yet another time bomb ticking away. As Dr. Kogler had put it, we had indeed been sitting on a barrel of dynamite, and it had already gone off. For Barry, it would not only be the end of the Vitaxin era. It would be the end of the eating era. He was only 12 hours away from having the feeding tube installed into his abdomen when Dr. Barone, the surgeon, reappeared at the doorway. He caught Barry by surprise as he was finishing off some ice cream.

"You can tolerate that?" he asked.

"So far so good," Barry replied.

"Do you mean to tell me that you have been having a full liquid diet here?" the doctor asked.

"Just in the last day or so," Barry said.

"Well, now, that really changes things!" said Dr. Barone as he tilted his head. "Have you ever considered having a stent?"

"What's that?" we both asked.

Neither of us had ever heard of it before.

"A stent is a prop that can be inserted into your duodenum. It will clear the passageway so that food can pass through. If you can tolerate what you're eating right now, you can probably tolerate a stent and continue eating real food. You'd have no need for the feeding tube."

His words sounded like magic! Never did we imagine this was even possible. From that time on whenever I saw Dr. Barone, it was with a halo around his head. Could things turn around so suddenly—and for the better, for a change? And why had no one mentioned a stent before? What if he hadn't appeared at that second, while Barry was in the middle of his meal? His eating days would have been history.

It turned out that this procedure could not be done at Sharp Hospital. In fact, it must have been one of the few procedures that could not be done at that hospital. According to Dr. Barone, only a couple of doctors in the region were capable of inserting a stent. It was a rare specialty. The doctor he recommended was out of the country. And the other was affiliated elsewhere, at the University of California at San Diego (UCSD) Medical Center.

After six days in the hospital it seemed that with the exception of a series of blood transfusions, little was being done. Barry's frustration was reflected by his blood pressure, which shot up by 100 points in a day.

"This could be your last Christmas," Dr. Pressman said. "You want to make it as special as possible. If you like, I can see to it that you have a single room for Christmas Day."

Barry and I glanced at each other. It was a kind gesture on his part, but not the kind of Christmas celebration either of us had in mind.

"I think we'd rather see Barry out of the hospital altogether by Christmas, don't you?" I asked. "Do you think that's possible?

Finally, on December 23, Barry was released. We stopped to visit a friend. Within a half-hour of arriving at our friend's house, Barry was on the telephone with Dr. Kenneth Binmoeller at UCSD. They briefly discussed his case and when the stent procedure could take place. They agreed on December 30.

I was so wiped out by Barry's latest hospital stay that I couldn't even imagine how—after all he had just been through—he could muster up the energy to call yet another new doctor. Had I been the patient, I would have already been at the end of my rope. But once again, as it had before, Barry's persistence paid off.

On the way home, we swung by Whole Foods in Hillcrest. Barry was so starved for decent food that he devoured his spicy tomato and basil soup. By the time we finally returned to Island Inn, we felt as if we had been to the moon and back.

On Christmas Eve, Barry's first full day out of the hospital, we took a walk around Seaport Village. The scene was eerily quiet. It seemed as if everyone had already finished their Christmas shopping and had left town. It was the calm after the storm. We attended Christmas Eve services with my family at their church in Cardiff-by-the-Sea.

> I felt very good being at church, not because I'm a
> religious person but simply because of the beauty of the rituals,
> the passion and gravitas of the priest, and the warmth and
> concern of the many parishioners, many of whom have known
> me for 20 years. It was a lot better than being in the hospital.

I, too, was grateful to be there. The church was an oasis for me as well. As we all knelt down to pray, I said a big "thank you" to God. By now I was convinced that a higher being was looking out for us. I was also eternally thankful for the prayers of so many parishioners surrounding me, and those of so many friends and family around the world. And I was relieved that, for the third time, Barry narrowly escaped spending Christmas in the hospital.

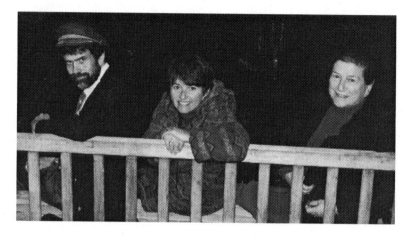

Christmas with Mom at Paradise Point, just days after Barry was released from the hospital. All he could eat was soup and ice cream. San Diego, California; December 1998. (credit: Harry Anthony)

The next day we joined my parents for an early Christmas dinner at a lovely resort on Mission Bay called Paradise Point. While Mom, Dad, and I enjoyed a normal meal, all Barry could eat was a bowl of butternut squash soup and chocolate ice cream. After dinner we took a boat ride on a Mississippi riverboat steamer. I was thrilled to be on a boat on Christmas day. With bright blue skies, warm temperatures, and a cool breeze, it seemed the perfect way to celebrate the holiday.

Later Barry and I stopped by another waterfront restaurant at Paradise Point where a lavish Christmas buffet was being served. Barry eyed each and every dinner item avariciously. Afterwards we spent a half an hour sitting by the restaurant's fireplace.

Today was nice being in a pretty setting and getting some fresh air, seeing the Christmas lights, and especially vicariously eating the buffet later in the evening and toasting my hands by the warm fire. It was a sensation I really enjoyed.

A few days later Barry went to UCSD Medical Center to have the stent endoscopically inserted by Dr. Binmoeller and a second doctor. They were in a large room full of bright lights, several large pieces of medical equipment, and a fleet of assistants.

Soon after we met them, one of the doctors told us, "You must have really good insurance! I know that HMOs rarely pay for a stent."

"That's just one reason why we're no longer in an HMO," I told him. And I couldn't help but think of all the millions of people who had no choice but to belong to an HMO, and what would have happened to them by now.

After the procedure was over, Dr. Binmoeller explained, "I saw lots of old blood plus some fresh blood. I saw many clots occluding the outlet of the stomach. Be careful. The tumor could grow through the mesh. It looks as if most of the tumor growth has been outside the stomach, and that it has grown from the outside to the inside. That's the one causing the problem. The tumor in the stomach probably did shrink with radiation. The problem is not so much the size of the tumor but its current location which is blocking the opening.

"You need to have frequent, small meals from now on. Watch out for breads, meats, and stiff vegetables. Even rice might clog it. You need lots of fluids to wash down small particles."

That morning Felicia arrived. In the evening the three of us walked over to the San Diego Convention Center where a spectacular New Year's Eve family celebration was underway. The idea was to get people off the roads on the holiday and keep them sober. The place was jam-packed and we could barely make our way through the crowds. Several bands were playing at once, revelers were dancing the night away, and the noise level was almost deafening. I began to wonder if going there was such a good idea.

As we wandered through the outdoor family area where hundreds of children were jumping up and down on inflatable toys, Barry suddenly said, "I'm feeling faint."

He was pale, weak, and drenched in sweat. His knees began wobbling, and he was on the verge of collapsing.

"Let's get him inside to the carpet so he doesn't hit the floor!" I said to Felicia.

He leaned on both of us as we carried him inside to a bench.

"Drop your head low, between your knees, Barry! That should get the blood circulation running." I said.

Then I ran to get some water from the refreshment area plus some empty boxes from one of the kiosks in case he vomited. Fortunately he didn't. We sat there for about a half-hour. First he was hot and dizzy, then cold and clammy. But he did not lose consciousness. Soon we took the elevator downstairs and walked the two blocks home. Barry rested as we watched the New Year's festivities on TV.

At midnight we saw coverage of the ball dropping 15 stories from Times Square West, the Aventine Center in La Jolla. At the same time we heard the sis, boom, bah of fireworks bursting over the waterfront. We ran to watch the display from our window. Behind the Marriott Hotel, shimmering streams of purple, gold, and red popped out of the sky.

On New Year's Day while the rest of the country was watching the Rose Parade, we drove over to Sharp Hospital. We waited there for three hours and met with Dr. Kogler. Although I thought that Barry would need a blood transfusion and be hospitalized all day, we learned that the previous night's near-collapse had resulted from an anxiety attack. The doctor prescribed Xanax, an anti-anxiety medication, and we were free to go. I was determined not to let the holiday pass us by. I drove out to Pacific Beach, where the three of us celebrated the new year at a restaurant overlooking the ocean. That evening we walked along Crystal Pier to watch the sunset.

Would Barry make it to the year 2000? Would we celebrate our 19th wedding anniversary, or our 20th? Could it possibly be a Happy New Year? After our tumultuous month of December—and our terrifying New Year's Eve—I was convinced that the answer was no.

CHAPTER EIGHT

Homeward Bound
(1999)

"It was the best of times. It was the worst of times."
—Charles Dickens

On January 4, 1999 we met with Dr. Kogler to discuss Barry's future medical treatment. Now that Vitaxin was behind us we were at a turning point. The choice was chemotherapy or nothing at all.

"The side effects could be quite severe and it may not be worth the trouble," Dr. Kogler warned us. "You will definitely begin bleeding more and you may have complications. And you have been bleeding a lot already. You'll need to spend even more days in the hospital. You'll need many more transfusions than you've had before.

"Your immune system will be drastically reduced, and you will be susceptible to infections. Usually we can control that but not always. What worries me most is the drop in the platelet count. Right now your platelets are high, but if they are reduced you will have difficulty forming clots.

"But you may decide to go for broke. In that case, we can give it a try and see what happens. If it goes well, it may even take care of the cancer on the lip, and that is about the only way we can tackle that. And if something goes wrong, we can always stop it."

I was convinced that we were finally at the end of our rope. After all he had just been through, the prospect of Barry having chemotherapy and more transfusions turned my stomach in knots. But Barry thought otherwise. The growth on his lip scared him. He had to do something lest it grow out of control. What if it grew so large that he couldn't eat or speak? And he had already had so many blood transfusions that they no longer frightened him. He was willing to go through more. Most importantly, he wanted to keep the cancer in his liver and abdomen at bay. So he decided to go ahead.

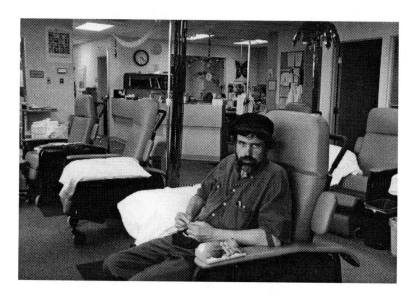

For roughly a year Barry required nearly two to three blood transfusions a week. Here he is in his favorite chair at the Sharp Infusion Therapy Center. San Diego, California; September 1998. (credit: author)

In January he began a new chemotherapy regimen of Adriamycin and Cytoxan. Adriamycin had a lifetime limit, and he would only be able to take a limited amount of it, as prolonged dosages could damage his heart. But that would be after some time. Those two drugs were selected based on the chemosensitivity studies on the tumor removed from his head in 1997. Another drug which seemed sensitive was VP16.

Before making our final decision, we ran the possibilities by Dr. Curley in Texas. He confirmed that Adriamycin and Cytoxan could prove promising.

Dr. Kogler's advice proved to be correct. Within just a few weeks of beginning the treatment, Barry was requiring blood transfusions one after the other, often three times a week. Sometimes he needed three units rather than two at a time. His hemoglobin level hovered in the sixes, and at times it dipped precipitously to the fours. Even though he had been checked every day, he was so weak one morning that spring that he could barely stand up to brush his teeth.

"I feel very weak and light-headed," he said. "My heart is racing just getting out of bed to go to the bathroom!"

"Forget about the teeth!" I said. "Do you feel well enough to get dressed sitting down?"

"Yes, I think I can," he answered.

As he slowly buttoned his shirt and zipped up his pants, I called downstairs to the front desk to ask for help. If we had had a wheelchair, now would have been the time to use it.

The executive assistant of Island Inn answered the phone.

"Barry is very weak and I need to bring him into the clinic", I told her. "Is there any way we can get a cart so that he can sit down and I can wheel him to our car? I'm afraid that if he's on his feet, he'll keel over!"

"Don't worry," she said. "We'll help you."

Within seconds the manager knocked on our door. He had brought up the office chair from the reception desk. It had wheels! What a terrific idea! He helped me carry Barry from the bed over to the chair, and then he wheeled him down the hall. He escorted us down the elevator and waited with Barry while I moved the car. What a lifesaver! At that moment I realized that we were probably better off living in an apartment than we would have been in our own house. At least here we had people to help us. As we drove towards the clinic I called the staff to ask for a wheelchair.

"We'll have one ready for you," Lisa told us. "Just call us when you're at the main entrance. Don't worry!"

I did so, and she was there on the spot. His blood tests revealed that his hemoglobin had dropped sharply from 6.2 the day before to 4.6.

A few weeks after beginning his treatment, Barry's hair and beard began to drop as well. Unlike four years earlier when his prior chemotherapy thinned his hair, this time it all came off. He found it smothered over his pillow when he got out of bed in the morning and all over the bathtub whenever he took a shower. What remained of his beard were a few stray wisps of gray and black hair which he stubbornly refused to shave off. It was part of his identity that he wouldn't let go.

In March CT-scans revealed that the tumors in Barry's liver had shrunk.

The radiation technologist who administered the test told Barry, "Boy, all I can say is that your liver sure looks a whole lot better than it did before! It looks like the liver of another person!"

By then it had been almost a year since we had had such good news. I could hardly believe it! I realized once again that Barry had been right. And all my doubts about his treatment had been wrong.

Throughout this period, however, Barry continued to vomit at least once every two or three weeks. We continued to carry the pink pails whenever we traveled by car. We also kept them stationed at our bedside. One of the more grueling episodes was when we returned from Julian, a scenic mountain town north of San Diego. After driving on the winding roads, Barry threw up violently. It had all come on too suddenly for me to pull over to the shoulder of Interstate 8. The stench was so strong that I opened all four windows and turned on the air conditioning full blast. As soon as I could, I took the nearest exit.

That spring when two good friends were visiting from Champaign, Barry, his mother, and I had gone to a festival in Little Italy. There Barry ate practically all that was being sold: pizza, pasta, a Sicilian oranchino, and gelato. I warned him several times but there was no stopping him. That evening while the five of us were strolling around the Gaslamp Quarter, Barry vomited violently all over the sidewalk in front of one of the Italian restaurants. I darted to get out of the line of fire. A few of the diners inside the front window grimaced and turned the other way. To them, he must have looked like a drunkard out of control. When a busboy came outside to see what was the matter, I felt terribly embarrassed.

"We're so sorry!" I explained. "My husband is a cancer patient."

"Oh, I see," he said. "Do you need any help? Even a glass of water?"

"No thanks, I'll be o.k." said Barry, as the busboy proceeded to spray down the sidewalk with detergent and water.

A similar incident occurred in the outdoor fast food court atop Horton Plaza. Once again Barry didn't make it to the restroom on time. The mess landed all over our table and gushed onto the walkway. Again I apologized to the maintenance staff. I began to worry that we were getting a reputation around town. People must have been saying, "Watch out for the guy with the Greek fisherman's cap! He spells trouble!"

Given the unpredictable nature of Barry's illness, I hesitated to go to plays and concerts lest this episode be repeated. I feared that we would be trapped somewhere in Row Q, Seat 12 when his urge to vomit would suddenly arrive. I could just see it spurting all over me and the other theatergoers in the middle of a play, stopping the performance midstream. Luckily enough, even though we continued to see a number of events, such a disaster did not happen. Yet clearly his body often roared out of control.

Despite all of this, for Barry, having the duodenal stent in his stomach made a world of difference. During the months that followed, he was able to eat normally once again—and actually gained 35 pounds.

Earlier that winter I had received an e-mail from one of my colleagues asking if I could teach a graduate seminar class on masters thesis preparation. I assumed that he was planning the teaching assignments for the following school year, since this spring semester was already underway. Much to my surprise, though, he was inquiring about the current term. Because it was a class where students conduct independent research, with period reviews and critiques by their professor, he suggested that I teach it on the Internet. Students could mail me their work and I could send it back to them with my comments. The university was willing to cover my expenses for two short trips back to Urbana, one early on in the semester and one towards the end, to meet with the class.

The prospect of earning some of my academic salary again was appealing. So was reestablishing contact with my colleagues and students. And I needed to take a trip home in any case, as again tax time was drawing near. Yet after all Barry's medical mishaps, the thought of teaching again scared me. Could I handle it? And did I even want to?

Although I hesitated to leave Barry alone even for a few days, I decided to say yes. It turned out to be a wise decision, and the class actually went better than I had expected. We established a computerized Web Board whereby the students read each others' draft thesis proposals and wrote comments on them. I responded to each of the students via e-mail. For this type of course, teaching by remote control actually worked. In February and April 1999, I took two trips to Urbana. I hadn't been home in about a year.

I was excited to enter the door of my office at 412 Architecture. Unlike last year, my office was just the way I left it, and no one else had been using it. All the mess had been put away, and the office looked better than ever.

My first day back in the classroom felt strange, however. Although by then I had been teaching for over 20 years, having been away from it for so long made me feel like a novice all over again. I'd jotted down a few notes in my appointment book to share with the students in class, but once I got there I found that either my handwriting was too small, or my vision had changed, for I had a hard time reading them. It also felt odd to be speaking one minute, and then have a room full of people dutifully writing down everything I was saying. After having been Barry's nurse, maid, chauffeur, and secretary for the past year and a half, I had forgotten what it was like to be a teacher.

At home, I was relieved to see that our house sitters had kept the place impeccable. By now there were actually two of them; the original house sitter had invited a friend to stay with him for a while, and in the meantime, he had moved in. House sitter #1 had stopped paying rent for his room near campus, he had stopped house sitting across the street, and now ours was his only abode. In fact, most of their worldly goods had been crammed into our small house. By now he had been living off and on rent-free at our house for a year and a half. During my stay in Urbana, I suggested that the two of them pay us $300 a month, enough to cover the utilities. Now that neither of them was paying rent elsewhere, I was beginning to feel exploited. After all, these two house sitters, one, a graduate student, and the other, a full-time campus employee, had access to an attractive three-bedroom house, while Barry and I were paying double housing expenses for over two years to live in a tiny studio. House sitter #1 agreed to this reluctantly, only after threatening to move out.

Seeing two other people's possessions spread around the house felt odd to me. It didn't feel like our house anymore. I finally came to grips with my discomfort by pretending that I was merely a guest at a Bed and Breakfast, one that happened to have traces of our former selves in it.

The other problem was that my house keys no longer worked. Apparently, because they had not been used for so long, the keys and the locks lost their grip on each other. I had discovered this the hard way—when I was almost locked out of my house late one night. Later I asked our house sitter to copy the set of keys I had lent him. Although he did so a few days later, the new keys were still defective. I would have gone to a locksmith myself, and in retrospect I should have, but I didn't have a minute to spare. Days later, when I was ready to return to San Diego, I drove with him to the airport in my car.

"Were you able to get another set of house keys made?" I asked.

"No, I was much too busy," he said.

"Oh, that's too bad," I said to him. "You know, it really doesn't feel good to be leaving my house knowing that I don't have a functioning set of keys to get back in. Promise that you'll make another set and send them to me right away. It's a good thing I trust you!"

"O.k.," he said. "And by the way, I'll need your car key to get home."

"Don't you have an extra one?" I asked.

"I guess I left it at home," he said.

"Well, promise you'll send me that key too!"

With that we said goodbye. As I watched my Honda fade off into the distance, I realized that not only did I no longer have access to my house. Now I no longer had access to my car. My stomach was churning as I stared in a daze at the airport ticket counter. And then it hit me: *My life had spun totally out of control.*

In May we celebrated our 19th anniversary in San Diego. While Barry had to remain in the clinic that morning for two blood transfusions, I was thankful that at least he did not have to spend our special holiday in the hospital. That evening he felt well enough for an anniversary dinner at the Reuben E. Lee, the Mississippi River steamboat where we had had our wedding reception. We sat at a scenic booth overlooking the harbor and the skyline. Although he made it through his meal, towards the end of it he began to feel queasy and hot. He disappeared in the restroom for about a half-hour, where he vomited his pricey dinner.

Around this time I asked Barry for his reflections. "What goes on in your mind when you are having a blood transfusion?"

I think about whatever book I'm reading at the time. Since I've come out to California, I've read at least 40 books. One of my favorites was David Denby's *Great Books* because it was a breath of fresh air in the longstanding debate over the canon and culture wars. That one stood out in large part for its intellectual honesty and its humility. Another book which had a powerful impact on me was Robert J. Lifton's *Hiroshima in American Memory* because for a quarter of a century I have been wrestling with some of these issues. There were times when I was reading certain books that I imagined myself being back at EIU thrashing out a couple of points at a graduate seminar. At times I even saw the faces of particular students before me, responding to particular arguments of mine, making arguments of their own, challenging certain assumptions. It wasn't the genuine article but it was the next best thing.

I've also read at least 60 plays here. I enjoyed David Mamet's *Glengarry Glen Ross* for its brutally honest portrait of greedy men on the make who will stop at virtually nothing to make it in our society. I especially was taken with two plays about Oscar Wilde, one of which I saw performed in Los Angeles, Moises Kaufman's *Gross Indecency*, and David Hare's *The Judas Kiss*. Both were exceptionally witty and imaginative dramas about an intriguing, not altogether sympathetic, individual. I've been a fan of Wilde's theater since I was a teenager, indeed since my early years in high school. I spent a considerable amount of time last summer reading the social protest dramatists of the 1930's, especially Sidney Kingsley and Clifford Odets. In addition I've read several of Edward Albee's plays, having long been an admirer of his since reading *Who's Afraid of Virginia Wolff?* The one that I found most searing was *The Death of Bessie Smith*. I've read a lot of Tennessee Williams since I've been here, a tiny bit more of William Inge. I particularly like those playwrights who are poets of pain.

"How does reading at the clinic during your blood transfusions make you feel better?" I asked.

If I'm reading a play, what makes me feel good is the plots, the characters, the dialogues, the themes, and the questions raised by the playwrights. For non-fiction, it is a cogent argument, a penetrating insight, a well expressed thought, an evocative phrase. Those are the kinds of things that get me going. I also like making connections among the various books I read.

"What else keeps your spirits up?" I asked. "Everyone asks me how you do it."

Seeing old films like the kind I grew up on, and going to see many of the plays that we've seen here. When I first discovered Garden Cabaret I was happy to see they were showing *Sunset Boulevard*, which I saw for the fourth time. And also I've really gotten into catching up on my old Hitchcock films. In a sense I've relived some of the happier moments of my childhood by virtue of being able to see these old movies that I would often stay up very late with my mother to watch back in the 1960's.

But mainly there was theater. *Death of a Salesman* was the most haunting play. It resonated with me because as an academic who was never certain he would not be a failure until just a few years ago, I could not help but empathize with the protagonist, Willy Loman. I also empathized with the lead character in *I Never Sang for My Father*, a youngish academic who had incredible difficulty relating to his father. Those were two of my favorite plays. I also found immensely stimulating Tom Stoppard's *Arcadia* because of the questions it raised about taste, criticism, historical investigation, scientific method, and the nature of truth.

And I've enjoyed the informal, off-the-cuff music we've listened to. It's been very eclectic. I felt relaxed and upbeat after hearing music, whether it was watching the Mainly Mozart performance here in the beautiful Spreckels' Auditorium or listening to Gershwin in the groves of Balboa Park.

Friends have always kept me going. I don't see too many friends on a regular basis here in San Diego. But I have my e-mail correspondence and my phone calls, and they both help. Most of all, I know that everyone is there for me: friends, family members, the extended family. I know that I can count on a large number of people to be there for me emotionally.

Time did not pass too slowly at the clinic because I spent at least an hour dozing off into never-never land. And when I was awake and not reading I spent a considerable amount of time talking to the nurses and fellow patients. In fact one of my nurses, Diane, dubbed me "the official greeter" of the clinic.

"Is there any particular philosophy that helps you get through this illness?" I asked.

Montaigne, a French wit who was noted for his aphorisms about life, love, and the human condition, once said, "He who fears he shall suffer already suffers what he fears."

There's an element of truth to it. I think that we can not help fearing, but we can certainly help what we do in the face of our fears. I've almost always tried not to let my fears paralyze me, but rather prod me to act more decisively than I would do otherwise.

By summertime Barry had eased into a routine of daily blood

drawings and regular blood transfusions. Because his treatment seemed to be working, and it was a conventional form of chemotherapy that could be administered anywhere, we realized that it was now time for us to return home. After two years away, it was time for me to go back to work.

It took us over a month to move out of our apartment at Island Inn. After having lived there for over two years, every inch of space was filled. We could barely see the floor. We tossed piles of papers, gave away extra clothes, and packed up box after box to mail home. Every time I looked around the room I realized that everything in sight except the furniture had to go. The scene was overwhelming. But all the while the calendar kept rolling. Our California adventure would soon be over.

By the time we left, we had visits from over 60 friends and relatives. Barry's mother alone had visited 10 times. In late July a group of friends from the Bay Area flew down to say goodbye to us. We ate a picnic lunch at Embarcadero Marina Park overlooking the harbor—much like our annual 4th of July picnics at San Francisco's Palace of Fine Arts—and dined in the Gaslamp Quarter, where we were entertained by a blues singer.

Around this time we decided that as long as Barry's health would permit, we would return to San Diego regularly. We had both grown to love the area. While it had always felt like home to me, after living there for over two years, it now felt like home to Barry as well. Barry could maintain his medical infrastructure there, along with his one in Urbana. With my academic schedule, we could theoretically spend a few months a year in California, back at Island Inn. My priorities had shifted. While I used to jump at the chance to earn a summer salary on campus, now I preferred to have my summers free.

"You only go around once," I thought to myself. "And you never know what the future will bring. So why not spend as much time as possible in such a beautiful place?"

Our last few weeks in San Diego were hectic. Moving took more energy than either of us could muster. I was absolutely exhausted. Some days I burst into tears, realizing that this chapter of our medical odyssey would soon be over. Another chapter was about to begin, but what would it bring? On the one hand, I had long feared that when we returned home no further treatment would be available for Barry, and he would be going home to die. But on the other, he was now on a form of chemotherapy that seemed to be working. Nonetheless memories of our two years in California kept spinning through my head.

I was dreading the moment when I would say goodbye to Mom and Dad. Now more than ever, I realized how much I loved them both and how much they had helped us during our most desperate hours. Years ago, if Dad had not sent us the article about David Cheresh and his work at Scripps Research Institute, we might never have known about Vitaxin. Without it, Barry would not have made it this far. And without Mom and Dad, I don't know how I could have made it either. They had been a steady source of financial support for both of us, enabling me to take so much time off from work. Without their help, even with my Family and Medical Leave, my sick leave, and Barry's meager disability salary, we could never have afforded to finance two households for over two years. More importantly, they had always been there for me. Whenever Barry was tied up at the clinic or at the hospital, I knew that I was always welcome at their house. Much to my surprise, all three of us maintained our exercise routine at the gym for a year. As a result, we were probably all in better physical condition than we had ever been before. They had become my safety net, my lifesavers. And I knew that I would miss them. When I watched their car disappear down Second Avenue, I struggled to hold back tears.

I also feared saying goodbye to the staff at the clinic. We had been there every weekday for the past year. In fact, we had begun to feel almost like Sharp employees, and all that was missing was a paycheck. We had even become friendly with the parking lot attendant, for whom we bought a small going-away present.

When I first saw the poster announcing the goodbye party that Mo had planned for us, I almost burst into tears. How grateful I was for all that they had done for us! And how thankful I was for all those San Diegans who had donated blood over the past two years. By now they numbered over 200. They were strangers whom I would never meet.

I feared that I would break down at the party, so I joined in the festivities early that morning and soon took a break. While Barry was having his final blood transfusion, I went for a final half-mile swim at the luxurious health club next door where I had treated myself on special occasions during the past two years. The pool and Jacuzzi always put me in another world, and the emphasis on health and fitness was a sharp contrast to the illness which surrounded me. Not only was Barry doing something for his health, but I was doing something for mine. And it sure beat sitting still for four hours. I was glad that I had taken some time out for myself, especially that day. I returned to the clinic refreshed.

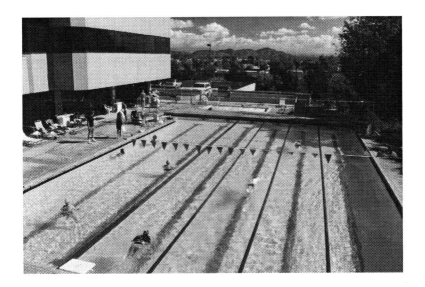

On several occasions while Barry was undergoing Vitaxin, chemotherapy, or blood transfusions at the clinic, I treated myself to a swim at this health club just footsteps away. While nurses were taking care of Barry, swimming helped me take care of myself. San Diego, California, August 1999. (credit: author)

Dan joined us at the party. It was hard to say goodbye to him. He had bent over backwards for us over the past two years as well—from bandaging Barry up after his head operation, to cleaning our carpet, to taking us sailing, to treating us for lunch, and visiting Barry whenever he was in the hospital. He had proven to us just how loyal a friend could be.

Michael, who had been Barry's nurse in the hospital at 8 North, also joined us for the party. I had contacted him only the night before and didn't expect to see him given such short notice, but he rearranged his schedule especially for us. It was a treat for us to visit with Michael while Barry was not in the hospital.

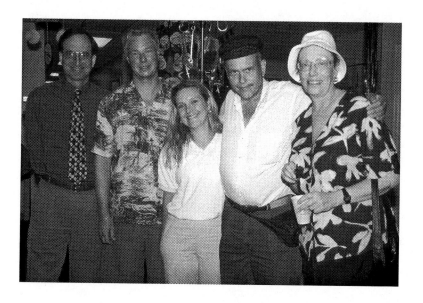

Daniel Shaw, Michael Drafz, Kelly Taylor, Barry, and Amy, another cancer patient at the clinic for our going-away party the day before we returned to Illinois. Amy passed away soon after. San Diego, California; August 1999. (credit: author)

Barry and I had ordered a pizza, and the nurses had brought in deviled eggs, empanadas, vegetables, and fruit. Fely, the phlebotomist, had prepared some Filipino lumpia, and Lisa, the nursing aide, provided some cookies that her brother had just brought from the Philippines. One of the other patients, Charlene, baked brownies. We munched away over the lunch hour and much of the afternoon.

The party made my stay in the clinic go faster than it ever had before. That is not to say that I was ever bored there, for I was not. Indeed, I had many pleasant and relaxing times there reading my plays and history books, talking with my mother, chatting with various patients and joking with the nurses. Also it was such an attractive environment that I was never depressed there.

That day, though, was something special. From the moment I walked in I felt as if I were the center of attention. And without trying to sound narcissistic, I guess that I was.

The nurses and the other patients alike made me feel that way. Interestingly, there were some patients that I had never met before who came up to me and said they had read about my story on the door of the Infusion Therapy Center. One of them, strangely enough, had the exact same cancer that I have. And yet he has lived with it for 16 years. I had thought I was doing well for a man in my position, but he may be setting the world's record.

Perhaps the most memorable part of the party was the end. I gave each and every one of the staff a hug. Some of them hugged me eagerly. One of my nurses, Diane, was a little reluctant to hug me.

"Oh no!," she said. "I've been dreading this moment all day long!"

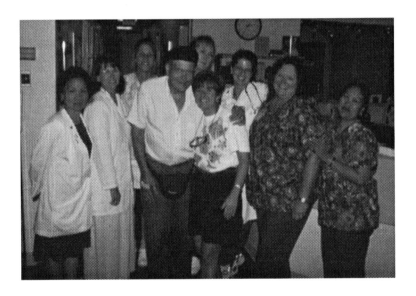

Our final goodbye to the medical staff at Sharp Infusion Therapy Center following Barry's last blood transfusion there. Several at our going-away party—including myself—were in tears but Barry was dry-eyed as usual. L-R: Fely Fluoresca, Patty Felts, Joan Hamrick, Barry, Diane Bradford, myself, June Childress, Margaret (Moe) Scarborough, Lisa Prado. San Diego, California; August 1999. (credit: Daniel Shaw)

Diane burst into tears. Mo grabbed a Kleenex and wiped her eyes. Lisa began to cry. And all day long I tried to prevent my own floodgates from overflowing. Ever since Barry's final packet of blood had stopped dripping, I knew the moment of reckoning had arrived. Long ago he had been King of International House. Now he had been King of the Clinic. Would he ever see all these kind people again? Or would I? Was this Barry's final goodbye? All these thoughts were swirling around my head as I gave each of the nurses a hug. But by then I, too, was overcome with emotion. I could barely see through my lens as I had everyone pose for a final going-away photo.

"Goodbye, Your Highness!" Lisa called out as we made our final exit through the waiting room door.

"Goodbye, My Liege!" said Barry.

———•·•———

At 4:00 the next morning we woke up to begin our trip home to Illinois. We had asked the receptionist to knock on our door, as by then we had no alarm clock and no phone, but he never showed up. I guess our own nerves woke us up. As we waited outside in the dark for the Cloud 9 Shuttle, guarding our six large suitcases, Island Avenue looked eerily quiet. It felt like the calm before the storm.

"This is it, Barry," I said. "Can you believe it? We're actually going home!"

———•·•———

Hours later we were on American Airlines flying over the Great Plains. I interviewed Barry during our flight. It was August 17, 1999, 11 a.m. Central Daylight Time.

> Right now I feel relaxed and tired from all the packing. I'm looking forward to seeing all my friends in East Central Illinois over the next few weeks. And to a somewhat lesser extent, settling into our charming home. I hope that I can get more work done on my book now that I'll have more time to devote to it than I did in San Diego. I will very much miss the Sharp Clinic to which I'd become accustomed over the past two and a half years.

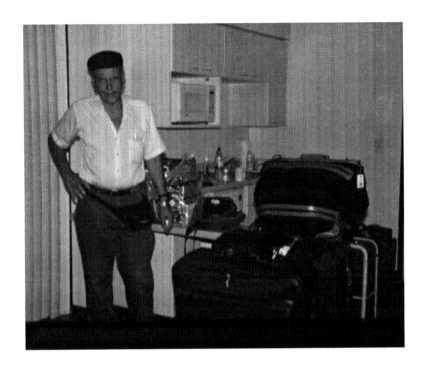

It took us a month to move out of our apartment at Island Inn, and by the time we left we were exhausted. Here is Barry at 4:45 a.m. the day of our departure with all our suitcases filled to the brim. After over two years in California we were finally returning home to Illinois. San Diego, California; August 1999. (credit: author)

In between talking and reading, my mind flashes back to yesterday, and in particular to the party that the nurses and staff threw for us. I remember especially the good food, the camaraderie, the well-wishing on the part of many fellow patients, and the laughter and tears of many nurses. It reminded me so much of my send-off by my colleagues just before I left for San Diego in the winter of 1997.

Naturally I feel somewhat uncertain about the future. I imagine and hope that I will readjust to Champaign-Urbana.

I am very much looking forward to seeing my friend, Mark Leff, today when he picks us up from the airport and welcomes us back. It will be nice to see one familiar and friendly face. Over the next few days I will look forward to hearing from and seeing people with whom I have been in touch for the last couple of years.

I cannot say what chapter of my life this is, but it definitely is a new one. I am eagerly anticipating the arrival of fall. For that is the one season that I have always treasured in the Midwest.

Over the next week or so, I imagine my mind will flash back many times to some of our favorite haunts in San Diego: The Horton Grand Hotel across the street from us (our extended living room), Mimmo's Italian Village, the neighborhood eatery where one could hear beautiful and memorable opera singing, the Garden Cabaret Theater where we saw some of my favorite old films and were treated far more warmly than we would be if we were at a conventional movie theater, the San Diego Pops concerts by the sea, the musicians playing at our nearby Seaport Village, the music we heard and the walks we took at lovely Balboa Park, the sights and sounds of the ever-colorful Old Town, the stunning Hotel del Coronado, the many new friends we made, and the incomparable piano player, Barry, at the La Valencia Hotel. Once he learned about my illness, he told us to come back any time, and he would play any song we wanted to hear. And he did—many, many times.

We arrived in Urbana that afternoon. Our longtime friend, Mark, met us at the airport and carried our six huge bags. It was reassuring to see a familiar face in what now felt like unfamiliar territory. As I watched Barry cross the threshold into our door, I couldn't help but recall watching him drive away so long ago, wondering if he would ever return. Now he did.

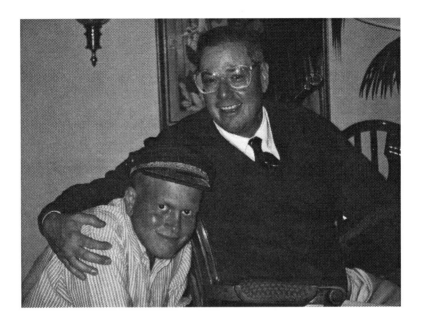

Barry Levich, the pianist at the La Valencia Hotel, offered to play whatever we wanted to hear. He was truly the peoples' pianist, and he knew thousands of songs. Music was therapeutic for both of us. La Jolla, California; December 1999. (credit: author)

Mark helped us not only with our suitcases but also with several large boxes that were awaiting us outside on our deck. They were the final shipment that we had mailed away from San Diego. Amazingly everything arrived intact. After Mark left we walked around our yard to reacquaint ourselves with what I used to call "our estate." As we reached the sidewalk a car pulled over. It was one of Barry's history colleagues.

"I thought it was you!" he said as he opened the window. "I can't believe you're back! And Barry, you look terrific!"

He grabbed him and gave him a bear hug.

For me, walking into 412 Architecture felt just as good as being back home. I relished having my office all to myself, and I realized now what a struggle it had been to work in our cramped quarters at Island Inn for so long. It took me days to go through all my office files and settle back in. Soon I plunged back into my teaching, research, and committee work. At faculty meetings the same voices echoed the same themes that they had two years ago, and at times it felt as if I had never left. I now had a full teaching load in the Design Division. I taught my environment and behavior seminar as well as my studio class, which I team-taught with a colleague. The studio met 15 hours a week and required a number of overnight field trips three hours away to East St. Louis, where our students were designing houses for low-to-moderate income residents. I enjoyed getting back into the swing of the semester again; however the heavy course load left me with little energy for much else. I usually left for work by 9 a.m. and did not return home until 8 p.m. after my seminar, often with a splitting headache. I worked 60 to 70 hours a week just to keep afloat.

My day began with a morning exercise routine, either a walk with my neighbors or a trip to the gym on campus where I worked out on a stationary bike and lifted weights. I forced myself to rise an hour earlier than usual to squeeze in that routine; otherwise the day would go by without it. After my year at the La Jolla YMCA, I had become addicted to exercise. I found that whenever I skipped my workout, I felt not only more tired but also more emotionally fragile.

Soon after we returned Anita, Barry's department chair—and another fitness fiend—stopped by to visit. She was waiting in our living room as Barry made his grand entrance.

We lingered over some cold drinks as she filled us in on the news of Barry's department. A few days later she hosted a potluck at her house to mark the start of the new school year. There Barry was reunited with all his colleagues. Within seconds he was back in his element, chatting away about history and politics while munching away on all the food.

In September our neighbors hosted a potluck block party where Barry rejoined our longtime friends from Pennsylvania Avenue. Carole had stopped by our house soon after we arrived, but Barry had not seen her husband, Tino, until the party. They gave each other a huge hug.

"You're a real fighter, Barry! You've got the will to live!" Tino exclaimed.

Several other neighbors who hadn't seen Barry in years marveled at his return.

The morning after our return Barry and I headed to Carle Clinic. Since he had last seen it, the Cancer Center had been remodeled and

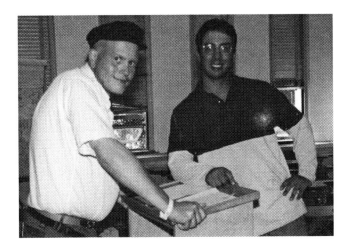

Barry back in his old classroom at Eastern Illinois University, with a former top student, Brent Cole. Here he felt a brief wave of nostalgia. Charleston, Illinois, September 1999. (credit: author)

looked much more attractive than before. When he told the staff about his need for daily blood drawings, they looked surprised.

"We've never had any patient need that here! We'll have to talk with Dr. Johnson. But if she says to go ahead, we will."

A few days later we met with Dr. Johnson. Her face lit up when she greeted Barry.

"I can't believe how good you look! It's great to see you! You're amazing! You're really amazing!" she said as we delivered our huge stack of medical records. "It will take me a while to get through this!"

In fact, Barry did look good. He had gained 35 pounds since January. Despite being on chemotherapy, which usually causes patients to lose weight, his stent was working so well that he could now eat just about anything. He had tried eating frequent, small meals for just a few days after the stent was inserted, but he soon graduated to regular meals. After so many months of eating only pureed foods, he was now in food heaven.

Dr. Johnson proceeded to treat Barry with the identical regimen that Dr. Kogler had used: Adriamycin and Cytoxan every three weeks, along with daily blood drawings and transfusions as needed. Barry continued to require blood transfusions about once or twice a week throughout most of the school year. And during our first week home, he actually needed four transfusions.

During that time we had a scare. One day we had been sitting out on our deck, and I noticed that sweat was dripping down Barry's brow and all around his Greek fisherman's cap. I followed him inside and upstairs as he headed to our bedroom to lie down. As he climbed the steps he began to sway back and forth. I stayed closed behind him in case he fell. By the time he made it to the top of the steps, he dragged himself to the bedroom and collapsed on top of our bed. It turned out that his hemoglobin had dropped precipitously and the next day he was transfused. I worried about being back in our house where the only bathroom was up a flight of stairs. What if he couldn't make it that far?

In the meantime, with 15 boxes and six suitcases to unpack, our house soon became a mess. It remained so for several weeks. At one level it was a relief to graduate from our 300-square foot studio to our 1400-square foot house. Yet since all but a few rooms were crammed with things, it didn't feel as if we had much more space. At night the neighborhood felt like a ghost town. While by day we could see lots of walkers and joggers along our sidewalks, at night, except for a few headlights here and there, Pennsylvania Avenue died down. It seemed so incredibly dark. We missed the commotion of the Gaslamp Quarter and the hustle and bustle of the city.

> When I first went home it was nice to see the house because it looked better than I anticipated. It was great to have more space. And it was especially gratifying to see our beautiful, colorful rug in our living room, one that I lived with for only less than a year. At nighttime it felt strange to go to bed and not to have a view of anything. It also felt strange to go to bed in such a dark room. I missed the lights of the Hyatt Hotel, the carriages rolling by underneath our window.

"There's no one to greet us when we arrive home," we often said as we drove up our long gravel driveway.

We missed the staff at the Island Inn reception desk who always said hello to us as we asked for our mail. And we had become accustomed to life as urbanites. It took us a while to feel comfortable in our single-family home and our serene neighborhood again.

At home we had work to do everywhere we turned. Our yard looked like a jungle, and six-foot high weeds filled our backyard. The paint outside our house was peeling and the west facade looked like a slum. Our gutters were falling apart. Our chimney was crumbling. The lights on our deck were out. The remote sensor on our driveway stopped working, and the darkness scared us whenever we drove in at night. Our electric garage door opener was broken, and despite all my weight lifting, our rickety garage door felt much heavier to me than before. Our door locks no longer worked. Our kitchen garbage disposal was broken. Our VCR was broken. Our basement was a mess. And the tape deck in my car was broken too.

One by one we tackled most of these tasks, but they were overwhelming. It cost us thousands of dollars to bring the house up to snuff and more often than not, the workers failed to show up on time—or even at all. We had to bring one of them to Small Claims Court, a frustrating process that took months.

We went on a massive clean-up campaign, giving away piles of books to the Urbana Free Library and box after box of clothes to a local charity. After living with less for two years, I resolved to rid ourselves of whatever we no longer needed. But this task, too, soon became overwhelming, and once I became buried in my schoolwork our clean-up campaign came to a halt.

"Now that we're finally back in Urbana, how does it feel?" I asked Barry.

During the fall I was going through my ritual of receiving blood drawings and blood transfusions frequently. I was comfortable in my new setting. The nurses were fine. I was able to hang out at my Espresso Royale café and see various friends there, and that felt just like old times. Plus I wrote two chapters of my book, one on the culture wars and another on the so-called Reagan Revolution. It was also nice to get back in touch with my Eastern colleagues, at a picnic, at a dinner, and at an event sponsored by the university, and at the annual Christmas party. I felt good being back on campus and seeing some of my history colleagues and friends. It was great to go to various architecture-sponsored events and occasionally go to music recitals and/or concerts. And it was wonderful to see our friends.

That year we were welcomed with a spectacular autumn. The weather was sunny almost every day and there was very little rain, except on a few nights when it rained just enough to make the grass and trees sparkle the next morning. The fall foliage lasted longer than usual, and we enjoyed watching our maple trees turn a brilliant yellow again. Even people who had lived in Champaign-Urbana their entire lives said it was the best fall they had ever seen. At Halloween the trick-or-treaters arrived just as they had done before.

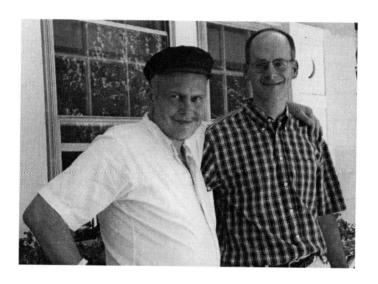

Gary Whitmer was one of our first friends to welcome us back to the Midwest, having driven out to see us from his home in Kansas City. He had also visited us in San Diego when Barry was first on the national news. Urbana, Illinois; September 1999. (credit: author)

Friends and family soon came to visit us from afar. In Champaign-Urbana and Charleston several friends entertained us, hosting us to dinner at their homes or taking us out to dinner. We were treated like royalty, and it was very spoiling. Spending time with our friends was the highlight of our return home.

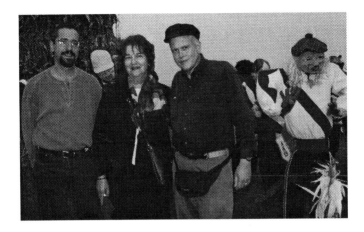

My cousin, Jack Rozos from Maine, and my aunt, Helen Rozos from Florida, visited us shortly after we returned home. The straw figures in the background were displayed at a local pumpkin patch. Arcola, Illinois; October 1999. (credit: author)

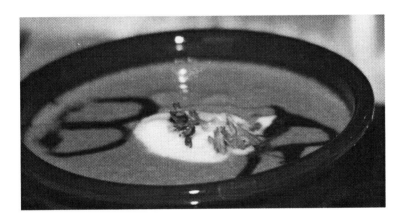

Now that we were back to a stove, oven, and full-sized refrigerator, Barry could enjoy cooking again. Here is his famous pumpkin soup with his initials dribbled in molasses. Urbana, Illinois; October 1999. (credit: author)

One of the other most rewarding aspects of our return was the ability to cook again. After lacking a real kitchen for two years, I had almost forgotten how. But Barry's memory never failed him. Within days he was preparing delectable dishes. As the aromatic flavors of Barry's cooking filled the air, our house felt like home once again.

I especially enjoyed getting back into a cooking routine which included most of the grocery shopping. I cooked some of my favorite dishes again, especially the old standbys: my pasta Or-Italia; chicken with orange mustard sauce; pork chops with apple cider, apple butter, pumpkin butter, and apple brandy.

On November 15 we celebrated Barry's 45th birthday at home with a small group of friends. It was a treat to finally have Barry back home for his special holiday. To commemorate his triumphant return, I had draped a colorful "Barry" sign— the same one that friends had hung in their house for Barry's tenure party three years before— over our fireplace. It lived on our mantle piece for the next year and made a scenic backdrop to the birthday photos.

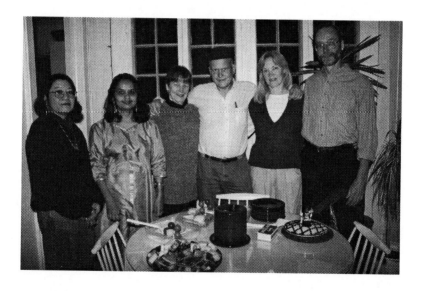

Celebrating Barry's 45th birthday, his first one at home in three years. L-R: Monica Chan, Amita Sinha, Norma Vyse, Barry, Diane LaBarbera, and Rich Nelson. Urbana, Illinois; November 1999. (credit: author)

That Thanksgiving Sharon and Reed invited us over, just as they had done years before. Amita joined us for dinner along with some other friends.

"Let's each think of something to be especially thankful for today," Sharon said. Soon each of us shared our thoughts around the table.

"I'm thankful to be alive," Barry said.

"And I'm grateful for the hundreds of people who have donated blood to keep Barry alive," I said. "I don't know who they are, but I often picture them lined up, block after block. Without them we both wouldn't be here!"

That Christmas we returned to San Diego for a month.

"It was very nice to feel the pleasant San Diego breezes and the warm California sun when I got off the plane," Barry said. "Plus I was looking forward to seeing all our friends and my associates at the clinic."

This time we were back at Island Inn but in a different room, #272. It had a small balcony which sat right atop the cafe. In the mornings the aromas of coffee and waffles wafted into our room. Every day we ate our breakfast outside on our two pink beach chairs, overlooking Island Avenue.

> Going back to Island Inn was in a sense, déjà vu. And I was very pleased with our room. Once I heard we were not getting the same old room, I thought we would get one that was very ordinary. But instead we were given one that was quite nice.
>
> I enjoyed the very pleasant weather and sitting out on our balcony every morning eating breakfast. It was also very pleasant to run into our old Island Inn friends, one of whom treated my mother and the two of us to dinner on New Year's Day.
>
> I was especially pleased to see my nurses and staff at Sharp Clinic. It felt almost as if I was returning to my old high school after being away at college for a semester. They were all very glad to see me, and I was very glad to see them. There was no adjusting for me because that, too, was my home away from home, almost as much as Island Inn.
>
> When I arrived at the clinic, one of the nurses, June,

spotted me out immediately, and shouted out, "Barry!"

And then all faces turned towards me and smiled. I was the center of attention. It was a very gratifying feeling to know so many people were happy to see me, and to see me looking so well.

Even Dr. Kogler was amazed to see Barry.

"I have never seen you looking so good!" he said. "You look much better than before you left. You've been living off other people's juices but you're doing alright. You did better on this chemotherapy than anyone expected. In retrospect I think it was the right decision."

"Even the protrusion above my upper lip was a pitiful shell of its former self," said Barry.

Later we visited John Gutheil, who had overseen the Vitaxin study, and David Cheresh, who had invented Vitaxin. Both had now become friends of ours, and they, too were excited to see Barry.

Our first afternoon back we went to one of my favorite hangouts, World Curry, in Pacific Beach, and had a wonderful meal. And then we took a long walk at Mission Bay and along the ocean. That was one of the highlights of our trip.

Another one of the highlights of being back was the Boat Parade in Newport Beach and seeing our friends, Sanjoy Mazumdar and Dan Stokols and their families, observing the beautiful Christmas decorations in the lovely Balboa Island homes, and eating at a fabulous restaurant which was one of our favorite haunts while we had lived in Orange County. I enjoyed the evening immensely.

Even though I'm not a religious person, I felt good about going to Midnight Mass in Little Italy. We had seen a play in which a couple of characters had gone to Midnight Mass in Little Italy. That in part gave me the idea. I went largely because I used to go as a kid. I find Our Lady of the Rosary particularly attractive. It was a traditional Christmas Eve mass. I can't say the sermon was especially memorable, but that's how I traditionally remember Catholic sermons growing up. I was struck by the ethnic heterogeneity of the parishioners, and how

crowded it was, because I had never seen it that crowded
before.

We celebrated Christmas Day in La Jolla with my parents and my
sister's family. Compared to last year's holiday, it was wonderful to see
Barry eat his entire Christmas dinner. By the time New Year's Day
arrived, several friends and relatives came to visit us.

Barry continued to have daily blood counts and transfusions
throughout our California trip, and his regular chair at the clinic was
waiting for him. Fortunately all his transfusions took place on weekdays
so he did not have to spend any weekends at the hospital. Since his
white blood counts were low, the nurses advised him to stay away from
crowds on New Year's Eve. Felicia, Barry, and I had an early holiday
dinner at Royal Thai, our favorite neighborhood restaurant, and strolled
about the Gaslamp Quarter. All the restaurants were decorated with
party hats and balloons in anticipation of the evening's festivities. In
order to protect Barry from infections, we left before the masses arrived.
We returned to Island Inn to watch 1999 turn into 2000 in a series of
ceremonies around the world. The mood everywhere was sheer jubila-
tion. Here is how Barry put it.

> I was glad to be able to watch the festivities on television,
> and it was fascinating seeing how other nations on the other
> end of the globe celebrated the arrival of the new century. I was
> struck by some of the smaller islands, in particular those
> outside Australia and New Zealand, and I found the Eiffel
> Tower celebration one of the most memorable.

As the clock struck 12, we heard the sound of fireworks out our
window, and we watched another spectacular display over the bay.

"Happy New Year! And congratulations, Barry! You made it to the
year 2000! To the New Century! To the New Millennium! I'm so proud
of you!" I shouted as we rang in the New Year.

I couldn't help but flash back to all the close calls we had had in the
past, all the times I feared we would never reach this day. It was a
milestone.

I was very happy to reach what many people regard as the New Millennium, even though the real New Millennium doesn't come for another year. My hope three years ago was to make it to the year 2000. Now it is to make it to the year 2001, and I think that's achievable.

I could not help but think about the numerous courses I would have taught were I in good health, courses dealing with the nature of American foreign policy in the wake of the Cold War, and the evolution of our party system in the 21st century, not to mention the various culture wars that I had both taught and written about in the past. How would they manifest themselves in the early years of the new century? No longer would I be able to discuss with my students the meaning of politics, past and present. I was more of a spectator than ever before, and that was a role I would have to get used to.

As the 20th century drew to a close, I felt exhilarated just to be alive. How many people had dreamed of reaching this day? How many people had we known who didn't live to see this historic event? Were they looking down on us, celebrating from afar?

Barry, too, reflected on the number of cancer victims he had known who didn't make it to the year 2000.

My first relative to pass away from cancer was my Uncle Joe in 1964. He was only 45 when he died and spent the last year of his life on a feeding tube. He was exactly the same age that I am now, and he had a feeding tube, which I came very close to having. His memory continued to haunt me. My grandmother, Jenny Pacelli, struggled 25 years with breast cancer. At that time surviving so long with any cancer was virtually unheard of. She died at the age of 68 after the cancer had spread to her bones. I remember her being in great pain during the last year of her life. There was also my Aunt Florence, a fun-loving woman who was consumed very quickly by a particularly savage form of cancer while in her 70's. In 1995 at age 75, my mother's cousin, Rita Thomas, also died of cancer. She had long suffered from pancreatitis, and in the last few months of her life she came down with pancreatic cancer. Her death shocked and saddened me because even though I had always known her to be sickly throughout a good chunk of her adult life, she was also a tremendously strong-willed woman who seemed to have a very healthy outlook on life—and death.

Since I contracted my illness, a number of other acquaintances, friends, and relatives succumbed to cancer. Marge Keith, a neighbor of ours whom I had gotten to know at Carle Clinic, and who still looked quite good in spring 1995, was gone by October that same year after a harrowing several months of treatment. Another neighbor of ours on Pennsylvania Avenue, Emma Koenker, would occasionally be in the clinic with me. She had only just become a teenager when she was struck by brain cancer. Emma's parents, one of whom was a colleague of mine, had done all they could for their daughter. In fact they had even gone to Chicago so that Emma could have an operation that was impossible to do in Central Illinois. But it was to little avail. Shortly afterwards, Emma went blind. Not long after she turned 14, she died.

Just two doors away from us, another neighbor, Severine Albarosse, had been battling ovarian cancer for over four years. Severine and her husband, Charles Stewart, who was also a colleague of mine, traveled to Chicago for her bone marrow transplant. And yet only a few weeks after the procedure, she learned that her cancer had returned and that she had only a few months left to live. This was an especially poignant situation because Severine desperately wanted to see her daughter, Laura, graduate from high school. She didn't make it nearly that far, as Laura was only in 8th grade when her mother died in her mid-40's.

Don Queller was a colleague of mine who had been battling cancer well before I was stricken. And he had the scars to show for it. In fact one of his cheeks was puffed out considerably and he wore a black patch over one eye. Don, who lost his wife to cancer, was in the corridor down the hall from me in fall 1995, when I had my stomach operation. I never did see him then though, because he died not long after I was taken off the operating table.

Our mutual friend from Greece, Thanassis Papazotos, was another cancer casualty. For a year he had been Kathy's office partner. We remember him for his incredible lust for life, but after four years battling a grisly form of intestinal cancer, he met an untimely death in his mid-40's.

The first to go from my California clinic was Danny, an engaging middle-aged businessman with a tremendous amount of energy and a very appealing sense of humor. We never got to know him all that well, actually, for he died within weeks of our meeting him and his wife, Marge. Then there was Herb Santos, an affable older man who always wore a baseball cap, short pants, and knee-length socks. Herb and his wife, Marie, were always very cheerful when I spoke with them. There was also Marie Williams, an attractively coiffed petite woman who always was accompanied by her childhood friend, Elleen. Elleen drove many miles a day merely to pick up Marie and take her to the clinic; Elleen lived near the Mexican border while Marie lived in Coronado. Marie often seemed worried about her situation. For one, her husband had Alzheimer's. And for another, she was losing weight, she was in a fair amount of pain, and was consistently fatigued. Finally there was Charlene, a dignified and highly intelligent woman whom I came to know during my final months in California. Charlene was the one who baked the brownies for my farewell party. I was especially touched by her death because she had gone out of her way not only to bake the brownies but also to give me a going-away card with some warm words of her own. I was also a little taken aback by her death because she seemed to be in the best health of all the patients I had met at the clinic.

Yet there were examples of hope. Perhaps the most striking was Stephanie Kaupp, an attractive and vibrant breast cancer patient who was finally told that her cancer had vanished. Kathy and I became close friends with her and her husband, Sandy.

I was struck by the fact that many of those who had died of cancer had actually been diagnosed well after I first came down with it. For instance, my sister-in-law's mother, Jo Lass, whom I had known since I was 17, was a vibrant woman in her 70's. The last time I saw her in Christmas 1996 she was the picture of good health. Two years later, around Valentine's Day 1999, after complaining of severe headaches and a slight limp, she was diagnosed with brain cancer. Within a month she was gone. This was quite a shock to all of us, for Jo had been a vital presence in the Riccio household in Arizona. It was especially devastating to her daughter, Maria.

Our brother-in-law's mother, Annie Smith, was another case in point. She died from esophageal cancer. My Uncle Louie in Florida, also in his mid-70's, was yet another. A year after Barry fell ill, he was diagnosed with inoperable bladder cancer and died two years later.

Ironically, each of these relatives worried about Barry's condition, and yet it was they who succumbed first. Our network of support had always been wide, a trampoline to catch us whenever we fell. When any of its threads withered away, we felt a profound sense of loss. A part of us was melting away, like a snowman in 80 degrees. And it reminded us of how fragile life was.

Though I was saddened by all their untimely deaths, at the same time I considered myself lucky to be alive. After all, I had been given the death sentence several times—and by reputable physicians at that. But I was not so naïve as to believe that this could go on forever.

To use the language of American politicians during the early Cold War, I saw myself as waging a battle of containment, not liberation. In other words, the best I could hope for was merely to prevent my cancer from growing— for a brief period of time. My aim was simply to stave off the inevitable, not to conquer the illness.

CHAPTER NINE

The Runner Stumbles
(2000)

"THE MIGHTY OAK WAS ONCE A LITTLE NUT
THAT STOOD ITS GROUND."
— ANONYMOUS

Before we left San Diego that January, we hosted a group from the University of Illinois for an extended field trip called Prairie on the Pacific. It was a way to bring students to see the revitalization of San Diego's downtown, a process that long fascinated me. I hoped to provide inspiration to these students, so that when they returned home they could begin to transform their own communities. I was thrilled to see Midwesterners discover the beauty of the Golden State. Their eyes lit up as we ascended the tram to the Getty Center. They were awe-struck by the Salk Institute, an icon that they had seen in all their architectural history classes. And they jumped at the chance to wear shorts and t-shirts in the middle of winter.

We returned to Urbana just in time for school to begin. This time I was teaching an overload of three courses, including a design studio and two seminars. I team-taught the studio with a colleague. Our class was working again in East St. Louis, and we traveled there three times that semester. It was a busy term for me.

Here is Barry's account of his winter of 2000:

> Most of the second semester was uneventful as far as my
> health was concerned. I continued my routine of virtually daily
> blood drawings at the clinic and I continued to receive
> transfusions at least once and sometimes twice a week.
>
> When I was not at the clinic, I spent a fair amount of time
> at a local café, which was a hangout for graduate students,
> professors, and wannabee intellectuals. There I would begin by
> reading *The New York Times* and follow that up with several
> hours of note taking from books on various aspects of post-
> 1975 America. This was for my textbook on that subject. I was
> beginning to fall behind, at least in my own estimation, but I
> wasn't pushing myself quite as hard as I would have in an
> earlier time because I did not want to add any more stress to
> my existence. On some occasions I would even write out the
> rough drafts of some of my book chapters. In addition I would
> come across friends with whom I would discuss public affairs
> and historical interpretations. Typically just after lunch I would
> walk for close to an hour just to get some exercise and fresh air.
> And this was pretty much my life up until early May 2000.
>
> A typical day at the clinic would involve my arriving there
> at about 9:30, having just chauffeured Kathy to work. I would
> wait just a few minutes for my blood drawing and then about
> an hour or so for the results. More often than not, I did not
> have to stick around to receive a transfusion, but I wanted to
> get the news as soon as possible. On days when I had transfu-
> sions, I would normally arrive at the clinic at about 9:30 or
> 9:45, take the pills which prevented an allergic reaction and
> which also caused drowsiness, and then start receiving blood.
> That process usually took about four hours for two units of
> blood. Sometimes it could take even longer. While I was
> getting blood I usually chatted with those who were sitting
> next to me and even got to know a few of them rather well. I
> would also read the newspaper and various books on history
> and related subjects. And I would take a nap for at least an
> hour.

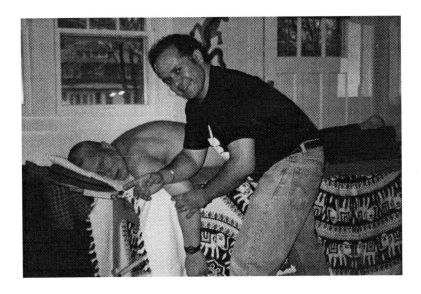

Kaizad Irani, one of my former students, made a house call to give each of us a massage. Urbana, Illinois; February 2000. (credit: author)

Once every three to four weeks I would receive chemotherapy. That was not as long a process as the blood transfusions, nor did they take my blood pressure on a regular basis as they did when I was receiving blood. The unfortunate thing about Decadron, a steroid drug I was getting, was that it kept me up at night. But since it was only about one night a month, it didn't bother me that much. The main drug, Adriamycin, would render me queasy for at least a day or two, although on that first day I would also have quite an appetite due to the Decadron. After the New Year, luckily, I did not throw up at all.

During that time I was working on yet another set of revisions for my book manuscript, *Designing for Diversity*. This was my fifth round of writing, and by now my enthusiasm for this project had waned. That spring I submitted the manuscript to the University of Illinois Press for what I hoped to be the final time. When I learned that the manuscript was accepted a few weeks later, I was relieved. My long nightmare was over, but another one took its place.

In May all hell broke loose. The cancer in Barry's liver was growing once again and it had now spread to one of his lungs. He had also reached the lifetime limit of Adriamycin. One more round of the drug would begin to damage his heart, so his chemotherapy was called to a halt. In fact, he had received far more doses of that drug than the typical patient, and even some of his nurses were amazed at how much he could tolerate.

Right around the time of my annual architecture awards banquet, during my last week of classes, Barry began to feel under the weather. During the next two days he caught a bad cold, and by the weekend it had spread to his chest. He was experiencing a tightness there that became more uncomfortable by the hour. He began wheezing. He suspected bronchitis, although I thought it was pneumonia, which he had had four times before.

On Monday, May 8, he was slated to begin a new chemotherapy regimen, high-dose Ifosfamide. We arrived at the clinic at 7:30 that morning since the chemo was to be administered 10 hours a day, five days a week, and we wanted Barry to have it as an outpatient. But once the nurses saw him, they could tell that he was in no condition to begin the treatment. He was having trouble breathing, he could barely talk, and he had great difficulty walking. At home, he could barely climb the steps to reach our one and only bathroom.

One of Barry's nurses was so concerned that she had him see a doctor and scheduled him for a chest x-ray immediately. Dr. Johnson was on vacation at the time, so we saw another oncologist who showed us the results of Barry's chest X-ray.

"Is there fluid in the lungs?," I asked. "Is it pneumonia?"

"No," he said. "It's not. I do see fluid around the lungs, but not in the lungs. It sure looks like bronchitis to me."

"Doctor, I'm scheduled to go to a conference in San Francisco tomorrow morning," I told him. "But I don't feel right leaving Barry this way. He can hardly breathe! It sounds like something pretty serious to me. If you think I shouldn't go, I'll gladly cancel the trip."

"You know what I think?" the doctor said. "With a day or two of antibiotics and decongestants, he'll be just fine. Go ahead on your trip, and don't worry. And if something does go wrong, remember: you're only a phone call away."

In retrospect I wish I had followed my own intuition rather than the doctor's advice. The next morning Barry drove me to the airport. After he dropped me off at the curb, he parked the car in the lot about 30 yards away. By the time I had checked in at the ticket counter, I walked back to the front entry to meet him. I found him seated next to the door. His face was gray.

"I could barely walk from the lot to get over here!" he exclaimed. "I'm completely out of breath!"

"This doesn't sound good to me, Barry. Stay right here, and don't move! Give me your car keys. I'll go move the car to that disabled space right in front of us."

As I walked back into the airport to greet Barry, I said to him, "You know, I really don't feel good about going anywhere right now. I don't think you should be left alone at home. You probably shouldn't even be driving!"

"But the doctor said I'll be o.k. Just a few days of antibiotics and I should be fine. Maybe they'll start working today. Go ahead and have a good time."

"Are you sure?" I asked. "If you want me to cancel my trip, I'll gladly do it right now."

"No, go ahead," he said. "And don't worry about me."

"Well then, be sure to check in a few times each day and let me know how you're doing," I said. "Take good care of yourself. I hope you're here when I get back!"

As my rickety propeller plane ascended above the cornfields, I had a sick feeling in my stomach.

"This trip is not starting out on the right foot," I said to myself. "Why am I doing this?"

By the time I reached O'Hare I grabbed my cell phone out of my bag and rushed to call two friends.

"I'm on my way to San Francisco for a conference," I told their answering machines, "But Barry's not doing well at all. He could barely walk from the parking lot to the airport. I'm really worried about him. Can you please look in on him while I'm away? And here's my phone number out West. Thanks so much!"

That evening friends took me out to dinner at International House in Berkeley. From the café we called Barry in Urbana.

"He sounds fine to me," said our friend Dean.

 In fact, I was forcing myself to sound stronger than I actually was. I spoke much more loudly than I would have normally.

 On Wednesday the situation continued to deteriorate. I was told at the clinic that my oxygen level was below normal. This disturbed me, for I usually had oxygen levels approaching 100%. Wednesday evening I went to the grocery store and rented a film, *Quiz Show*. I saw only the first half of it that night, as I grew tired and it was late. Needless to say, I assumed I would pick up the second half the following night. But there would be no following night, at least not on 309 West Pennsylvania.

 The next morning our neighbor, Carole Rebeiz, drove me to the clinic where I had an echocardiogram. The cardiologist immediately informed me that I would have to have emergency heart surgery.

 I was shocked beyond belief. I did not like the idea of my heart being operated on. As it turned out, the heart itself would not be touched. Rather the game plan was to carve out a so-called pericardial window just around that organ. The objective was to drain fluid from the pericardial region. The reason this had to be done was because the fluid buildup in that area was literally crushing my heart, causing me not only to gasp for breath but to turn gray.

 I asked the cardiologist if the surgery could take place on Monday rather than on Friday, which is when he wanted to have it done. That way Kathy would be back.

 He quickly responded, "We can't wait until Monday!"

 Later that afternoon I met with Dr. Johnson, and she informed me further of the gravity of the situation.

That Thursday afternoon I had returned to my hotel room in San Francisco to take a break from my conference. Soon after I opened my door, I saw my telephone light flashing.

"You have six messages," the automated voice told me.

Upon hearing those words, that terrible feeling in my stomach surfaced once again. The first few messages were from some old friends whom I had been planning to meet for dinner on Friday.

"Perfectly harmless," I thought to myself. "Maybe nothing is wrong after all."

But then I heard another voice, one that I never expected to hear in the Cathedral Hill Hotel, of all places. It was Dr. Johnson:

"Barry is about to have emergency heart surgery tomorrow at Carle Hospital. You need to come home right away."

My hands were shaking as I replayed her message, just to make sure I heard it right. Then I heard one more voice mail, this time from Barry. While simply knowing that he could speak on the phone was reassuring, within seconds I exploded into tears.

I frantically began opening the dresser drawers and packing up my suitcase, preparing for a quick exit. My clothes were still strewn all over the bed when I realized that I had more work to do. I called up my student who was down the hall and asked him to leave notes for my colleagues, canceling my participation for the rest of the conference. Then I left messages for two friends canceling plans for dinner that evening, and informing them that I was unable to serve as moderator for our two sessions the next day. I called my friend, Colleen, who worked a few blocks away, and explained what happened.

And then I called American Airlines. Despite my plea for help, a surly agent insisted on charging me full-fare. I argued with her several times before speaking with her supervisor. It turned out that all flights to Chicago were booked, and the soonest I could escape was first thing in the morning at 6 a.m.. Even so, I wouldn't get home to Urbana in time for Barry's operation that morning. But there was nothing else I could do. Within a few minutes, Colleen arrived.

"Are you alright?" she asked. "What can I do for you right now?"

"You know, I really need to go and take a walk," I told her. "I think I need some fresh air!"

That evening Colleen drove me out to Baker Beach where we took a scenic walk near the Golden Gate Bridge. The wind was blowing fiercely and it was chilly, but it felt great to be outside. The next morning at 4:30 she was at my hotel lobby to drive me to the airport. I could not have asked for a more loyal friend.

What was Barry's reaction to the sudden turn of events?

I was a little stunned at this point, but I was also preoccupied with trying to breathe. So consequently I may not have been quite as worried as I might have been under other circumstances. In any event, I phoned Carole and asked her to pick me up, drive me home, and then come back for me when I called her shortly afterwards to take me to the hospital for the operation. The doctors and staff would have preferred that I stay in the hospital. But I wanted to pick up a few items such as a toothbrush and a bathrobe and some clean underwear. In addition, I had left the house in somewhat of a mess and I did not want it to be in that state when Kathy returned home. I had to wash and dry the dishes, make the bed, and sort out the mail. It took me longer than I anticipated to clean up and gather my necessities because I was so out of breath that I had to stop and sit every now and then. Getting up the steps was a formidable task. In fact, once I got up the steps I had to lie on the bed for about 10 minutes. In between doing my errands I left a message for Kathy at her hotel, following up on what Dr. Johnson had said earlier. Just before Carole picked me up, Melissa, the nurse, called to find out where I was, and to make sure I was o.k. I told her that I was fast on my way there.

Checking in took about an hour, but my neighbor stayed with me during that period of time. Indeed, she was with me until I got to my hospital room. She said she'd be back the next day before I had the surgery. I had a very pleasant nurse and I was relatively comfortable that first night. That evening I received a blood transfusion. Because the procedure took so long, I wasn't able to fall asleep until the wee hours of the morning. Only a few hours later I met with the surgeon, Dr. Michael Colla, who seemed to be very knowledgeable. At this point I wasn't really afraid of the surgery and I was somewhat looking forward to being put to sleep for a few hours.

Shortly afterwards my neighbor, Carole, came to see me in my room. And not long after that, she, a nurse, a transporter and I all went to the operating area. Carole spent nearly an hour with me. By the end of that period the relaxing medication that the anesthesiologist had given me was showing its effects. I vaguely remember saying goodbye to Carole and going into the operating room, being strapped down, and being told I was about to be given the major anesthetic.

The next thing I knew it was about four hours later. The operation itself had only taken about 45 minutes, but I was so heavily sedated that I simply did not wake up until well after it was over.

While my flight to Chicago that Friday was uneventful, the rest of the trip was a nightmare. Due to a ferocious series of thunderstorms, my three-hour layover at O'Hare turned into five hours. I spent a good part of that time on the phone trying to track down Barry's doctor. Eventually I was relieved to learn that the operation was over. Just when I began to feel my nerves calm down, I heard my name broadcast over the loudspeakers.

"Would Passenger Kathryn Anthony please come up to the ticket counter?"

After making my way through the crowds, I asked the agent what was the matter.

"You were the last passenger signed on to this flight, and we need you to give up your seat," he told me. "This plane is oversold. We can offer you a free rental car to drive to Champaign. Otherwise we can put you on the next flight out later this evening."

"You can't bump me, sir," I told him as I felt my blood pressure rising once again. "My husband is having emergency heart surgery as we speak. I've got to get there right away. Here's a fax from his doctor."

With that he called out the next name. No way I was going to drive a strange car through a thunderstorm in Chicago's rush hour traffic, especially given the state I was in. By now I was so exhausted that I could have fallen asleep on the spot.

Finally the storm appeared to have cleared and we entered the small propeller plane to begin our journey to Champaign. The air conditioning was not working, the temperature and humidity were in the 90's, and everyone was drenched. The plane was packed with families headed for the University of Illinois graduation ceremonies that weekend.

When we reached our cruising altitude, things only got worse.

"Due to the short duration of this flight, we will have no beverage service," the flight attendant announced as we boarded.

But I knew what that meant. The storm that had passed through Chicago was now right in front of us. On both sides of the plane, streaks of lightning darted across the skies, and soon we were caught in the turbulence. We rocked and rolled, bopping up and down like a top.

As we continued our roller coaster ride, I feared that we would come crashing down from the skies.

"Why can't we live in a normal place, without these rickety old planes?" I thought to myself. "Barry's just escaped death—all too narrowly— and now my life is in jeopardy too. This is too much excitement for one day!"

When we finally hit the ground at Willard Airport and escaped from our chamber of horrors, I was relieved. But the skies still looked ominous. I bolted out to the curbside, searching for a shuttle van or a taxi, but found neither. I waited for 10 minutes and still none arrived. So I called our friends, Diane and Rich, who lived close to the airport.

Rich answered the phone. I described in detail what had happened and asked if he or Diane could give me a ride home.

"There's a severe storm warning out, and we really shouldn't be going anywhere. I just heard it on the radio," he said.

"In that case, don't worry about it," I told him. "Tell Diane to stay home."

"You know what?" he told me. "I think that while we've been on the phone, she's already on her way."

With that I began moving towards the front entrance of the airport. Then I heard an announcement over the loudspeakers.

"A severe thunderstorm warning has been issued for Champaign County. All passengers and staff must clear the gate area. Stay away from all glass. Gather downstairs behind the escalators until the warning is lifted."

But I couldn't heed the warning, because now Diane was risking her life to come and rescue me. So I waited outside next to the huge glass windows, hoping they would not come crashing down.

When I saw Diane's car pull up to the curb a few minutes later, I said to her, "Life saver!"

As we drove north down Neil Street the rain began to fall. First it was a steady stream, then it turned into buckets, and we could hardly see out the windshield. By the time we reached our driveway, the streets were almost flooded. We dashed into the house and I rushed to the phone to call Barry.

In the meantime Diane had turned on our radio.

"The National Weather Service has issued a tornado warning for Champaign County. Take cover immediately," said the radio announcer.

Diane and I ran to our basement, taking the radio with us. We huddled there for 45 minutes until the warning had been lifted. By the time I reached the hospital, it was already 8 p.m. I found Barry looking pale and weak, with those fluorescent lights shining on him, just as they had been after the ill-fated surgery in Houston years ago.

"You made it, Barry! You pulled through yet another operation—this time #6." I said as I greeted him. "We didn't think I'd be back so soon!"

After all his prior operations, I had never taken his photograph. I had always preferred to remember him as his normal self, not as a hospital patient. But this had been such a harrowing journey that I wanted to commemorate the grand finale. I had one frame left in my film, so I asked his nurse to shoot a photo of both of us. We sat and chatted for a few hours, but by 10 p.m. my eyes started drooping, and I headed back home.

The next morning, before driving back to the hospital, I soaked in a fragrant bubble bath, something to which I treat myself about once a year. Slowly but surely my head began to clear. Barry, though, was not feeling any better.

On Saturday, Kathy and I spent more time together. But my breathing did not really improve. Apparently some of the fluid from my heart, which was still being drained out, had migrated to the region around the lungs. So I was given Lasix and a nebulizer, a machine that sprayed a mist allowing me to breathe. I was also required to put on an oxygen mask. This mask was rather large and unlike any I had worn before. It felt slightly uncomfortable, but I could breathe better with it, so I didn't complain.

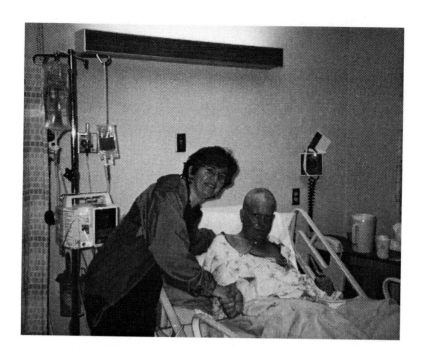

The two of us at Carle Hospital after Barry's emergency pericardial window surgery. Just hours before I had flown in from California through a severe Midwestern thunderstorm. Urbana, Illinois; May 2000. (credit: unknown)

On Sunday the tubes that had been draining the liquid from my heart were removed. That was only somewhat painful. About two liters of fluid were taken out. But because I still had so much fluid around the lungs, another set of tubes was inserted into that region. I was awake for this procedure. Luckily, the only real pain I had felt at that point had been from the urinary catheter, which had left me a bloody mess. And its removal was especially excruciating. I had had many of them over the years, but I never really got used to the experience.

That day Barry had a series of tests to determine how much of the area around the heart had been cleared of the fluid. As the nursing aide wheeled him around the maze of corridors and elevators, as he was jerked in and out of the X-ray room, and as the doctor ordered more and more X-rays, the severity of his illness hit me once again. Here was Barry—the vibrant, healthy man I married almost 20 years ago— reduced to a shriveled up figure, stooped over in a wheelchair. He had lost several pounds from the surgery alone. His head was still scarred severely from his operation three years ago. Except for a few goat-like gray strands protruding from his beard, his hair had all disappeared. And now his face was obscured by the oxygen mask. I felt so sorry for him, and yet there was little I could do except stand and watch.

Ironically, that Sunday was graduation day on campus. Since I was supposed to have been at my conference in San Francisco, I hadn't planned to attend the ceremonies. I hadn't ordered a cap and gown, and I hadn't reserved a spot in the faculty line-up. But now here I was in Champaign-Urbana, and for a few moments off and on that weekend, I felt as if I should be there. I dreaded bursting into tears in front of all the happy grads and their families. Instead, that morning I biked out to Meadowbrook Park where I enjoyed the springtime flowers. I talked to no one. By the time I visited Barry at the hospital later that day, I felt much better. But he would soon feel much worse.

> By midweek I was told I had to have something called a pleurodesis done to me, a procedure involving gluing the chest wall to the lungs. This entailed inducing me with pleuresy, and I did not expect it to be too painful. Unfortunately, however, it was agonizing. The pain I experienced in my back was excruciating. I was not mentally alert enough at the time to know exactly what the doctor's assistant and my nurse were doing, but the whole process took one hour. And during that period of time, I sweated bullets. Luckily I did catch up on my sleep afterwards.

I had called from my office to speak with Barry that afternoon. When another voice answered the phone, I was shocked. It was Barry's nurse.

"Barry can't talk right now," he said. "He's not doing real well. He's in a lot of pain."

His words sent shivers down my spine. Once again I felt so helpless. But by the time I visited Barry a few hours later, the worst was over.

Thursday was an eventful day. There were two tornado watches: one in the morning, and one in the evening. During the morning tornado watch, I was nearly evacuated from my room.

When one of the nurses was about to move me into the hall, another one warned her, "Don't do that! Don't disconnect him! If you do, his lungs will collapse!"

So they merely moved me to another side of the room, away from the windows.

That evening there was another scare. This time, however, I was actually evacuated from the room because I no longer needed that machine, and I no longer needed an oxygen mask. Kathy and our friend, Norma, were visiting that evening and were struck by the vast number of patients that were sitting calmly in the hallway for well over an hour. I wasn't too worried about it, because I knew I would be going home the next day.

Friday did indeed prove to be Emancipation Day. Kathy picked me up in the early afternoon. I was stunned by how cool the weather had turned, because it had been very hot when I went into the hospital just a week earlier. When we got home, our housekeeper, Pam, greeted us. I was still too tired to talk much, so after a glass of cold water, I went upstairs and took a lengthy nap. That evening one of my friends from Oregon called me. Kathy made the first good meal I'd had in over a week, a Chinese shrimp stir-fry dinner. We also started watching the second half of *Quiz Show,* which I had checked out a week earlier. The next few days I basically rested, saw videos, and did a little bit of reading. When I was in the hospital, though, while I did not do as much reading as I would have liked, I did manage to get through a funny and touching David Lodge novel entitled *Paradise News.* It was about a group of Brits visiting Hawaii and the various relationships among them. So taken was I with that novel that when I

got home I began to read another of his works, *Changing*
Places, a satire on two professors who exchange positions, one
in Berkeley and one in Birmingham.

Soon after Barry was released from the hospital after his heart
surgery, he began experiencing severe pains in his anal region—a literal
pain in the ass. No matter how he sat or how he lied down, he couldn't
get comfortable. Having had a history of hemorrhoids, he suspected
that they were the culprit. But it turns out that his discomfort was
caused by a chronic fissure, one that may have been exacerbated from
his eight-day hospital stay and spending so many hours in bed. Ironically, the doctor who would perform the outpatient surgery was Dr. Lyn
Tangen, the surgeon who had first operated on Barry almost seven years
ago.

"You've had a rough time since I last saw you, haven't you?" he said.
"But it's good to see you again. You're a real fighter! I can see that!"

We spent a good portion of the day scurrying about the hospital
from one appointment to another, filling out what seemed like reams of
paperwork. It all seemed so ridiculous in light of the fact that just days
ago, he had been a patient in the same place. After all, wasn't all his vital
information stored on the computer? To top it off, as we were leaving
our first appointment, the administrative staff produced a two-foot pile
of file folders.

"You need to carry these with you for all your appointments today,"
they told Barry. "These are your medical records."

Within minutes Barry and I were winding our way through the
hospital corridors. The patient was walking at a brisk pace, with his
medical records piled high atop the wheelchair in front of us. When we
reached Dr. Johnson's office the nursing aide asked Barry to step on the
scale.

I interrupted, "Wait a minute! Would you mind if we weighed
these too? I'm really curious to see this."

"No problem," she said.

Together we placed the mountain of files on the scale. They
weighed 24 pounds! I shouldn't have been so surprised. After all, by
now his medical files, hospital bills, and all my notes about his illness
had spread to over three large file drawers at home.

Two days later Dr. Tangen performed the procedure on Barry's anus, and I was back in the surgical waiting area of Carle Hospital, as I had been years before. Once again, I brought in my CD player to drown out those stupid game shows blaring on TV. And once again, I watched all the wiped-out family members and friends of patients, anxiously awaiting to hear their names called. I relished the fact that this time Barry's surgery was only 15 minutes, plus a few hours for recovery, and I could take him home right away. At least for the time being, this was not a matter of life and death.

But in the meantime, more than the surgical procedure had passed. The night before was an even more significant event for both of us.

> That evening Kathy and I celebrated our 20th anniversary with several of our very best friends: Norma, who was at the hospital the night of the tornado evacuation; Diane, who had applied cold applications to my forehead after my third operation in 1995; Amita, a longstanding friend who had visited me in the hospital many times before; and our neighbors Carole (who had not only driven me to the hospital but actually stayed around to hear the results of the surgery) and her husband Tino. We ate at Silver Creek, one of our favorite restaurants, which had charm and generally quite good food. Virtually everyone commented that I looked amazingly well considering what circumstances I had been in just a while before. All in all, it was a most enjoyable evening—perhaps a fitting end to yet another messy chapter in my saga, and the beginning of yet another phase in this long medical odyssey.

As we toasted around the table, I couldn't help but think how often I had feared that we would never reach this day. Images of the past seven years flashed through my mind. I wouldn't wish them on anyone. In many ways, they had been seven years of hell: seven operations, hundreds of medical appointments, hundreds of blood transfusions—and all those gruesome vomiting episodes. I had seen enough blood and guts to last a lifetime.

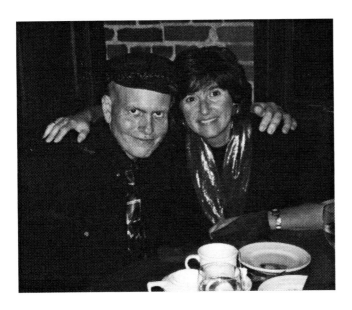

Celebrating our 20th anniversary. At times both of us doubted we would reach it. Urbana, Illinois; May 2000. (credit: Norma Vyse)

And once again, the memory of all those countdowns flew by me. Countdown until we drive away to Minnesota. Countdown until we drive away to Texas. Countdown until we fly away to Detroit. Countdown until Barry drives away to California. Countdown until we return home to Illinois. And just this month, while rushing home from San Francisco, another countdown too.

In fact, by this time Barry had spent a total of 72 days, or two and a half months of his life, in a hospital. For 296 days, almost 10 months of his life, he had been an outpatient in a clinic. And I had been at his side for most of them. Miraculously, he never complained. How fortunate was I still to have Barry as my husband after 20 years. My love for him had grown exponentially with each passing year—and living in the shadow of death had brought us even closer.

I would not wish even on my worst enemy the financial havoc that this illness left behind. By this time, our out-of-pocket medical expenses had totaled almost $54,000, about $9,000 were still in question, and no doubt we would eventually pay thousands more. Our preferred provider

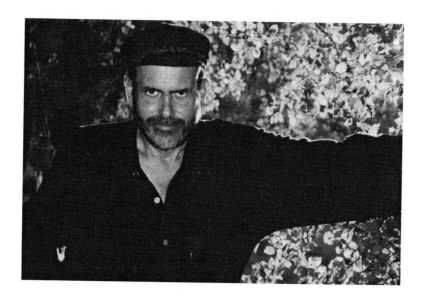

No doubt that Barry outlived all his doctors' expectations through his enormous patience, persistence, and perseverance. Lakeside, California; July 2000. (credit: author)

organization insurance had paid $564,000 to keep Barry alive, and I could only imagine what would have happened had we not had such excellent coverage. All our life savings would have been wiped out years ago. Had we remained in our HMO, our expenses would have been far fewer, but the bureaucrats would never have approved all our out-of-town travel, all those blood transfusions, and all those daily blood drawings. Without question, under the so-called care of an HMO, Barry would have been dead long ago.

So many times during our stay out west I had pleaded with him, "Barry, so many friends have urged us to get our story on paper. We've simply got to write our book. Now I have time, but once I'm back at work, whenever that is, I probably won't. It's now or never!"

"But hardly anyone will be interested in our story," he said. "I'm no different from anyone else."

"Oh yes, you are! You're special! Look at how far you've come!" I reminded him.

"Oh no, I'm not," he said. "I'm just a desperate man in desperate circumstances. I've been dangling at the precipice, trying to keep myself from falling. I did what anyone else would have done."

"But you're wrong, Barry! You've done much more than that," I said. "You've outlived all your doctors' predictions in large part because you've done what most other people would *not* do. Even I would have given up long ago. Someday you will be gone, but your spirit will live on. Others who never got a chance to meet you will know about you too.

"And think of all those people who will be diagnosed with cancer and other life-threatening illnesses, all those stuck in rural areas or trapped in HMOs who believe they have no way out. And all those who will undergo novel treatments like you did. They'll want to contribute to science just like you. They, too, will put their bodies on the line. And they might be on the verge of getting tossed out of their protocols, just like you. Think of their families and their friends—people who will experience the emotional roller coaster ride that we've both been through. They need to hear our tale. They need to learn to take their lives in their own hands."

The cancer had hit us like an earthquake, and we were still reeling from the aftershocks. But the patient was still here.

And as I had often said, "As long as we're still all around to discuss it, it can't be all that bad."

And so this book began. No longer was Barry simply a historian. No longer was he simply a professor, an author, and a playwright. No longer was he simply my husband and my best friend. No longer was he simply a cancer patient. He had made medical history. He had broken new ground. He was a pioneer.

And no longer was I just the wife of a sick man, with that big "C" etched across my forehead. No longer was I just a professor, a researcher, and a scholar who could write only about architecture. Writing our medical odyssey forced me to pry open that lid, to burst out of that box. It was something I had been longing to do. Now I could write about life. It was a new awakening.

No doubt our normal lives had been robbed from us, and we would never get them back again. Yet had we lived 20 or 30 years ago—or in many parts of the world today, for that matter— most of the treatments Barry had received would not have been possible. Had we not traveled to Texas to the MD Anderson Cancer Center in 1994, we would never have met Dr. Curley, who proved to be our lifeline many times over. Had our neighbors not informed us of photodynamic light therapy, had Barry not called Dr. Fromm, and had we not traveled to Michigan in 1995, we would not have had yet another reprieve. Had Dad not sent us the article in 1996 about the promising studies at Scripps Research Institute, and had Barry not driven out to California in 1997 to participate in the Vitaxin protocol, his life would not have been prolonged by almost two years. Had Dr. Barone not magically appeared at our hospital room doorway in 1998, and had Barry not contacted Dr. Binmoeller at UCSD, Barry would have been reduced to life on a feeding tube. Had Barry not been willing to risk more rounds of gut-wrenching chemotherapy, he would not have been sitting at this table. Had 350 strangers not donated blood for all his transfusions, we would never have reached this milestone.

And had our multitude of family and friends not been there for us, had I not been able to take a leave from work, and had I not become a fitness addict, no doubt I would have cracked under pressure. At times I had come close. But Barry never faltered.

As I watched Barry chatting away with our neighbors, I smiled. For the past seven years we had been running for our lives. And we would keep on running.

EPILOGUE
(2000-2001)

"HE WAS MY NORTH, MY SOUTH, MY EAST, MY WEST,
MY WORKING WEEK AND MY SUNDAY REST,
MY NOON, MY MIDNIGHT, MY TALK, MY SONG;
I THOUGHT THAT LOVE WOULD LAST FOREVER: I WAS WRONG..."
—W.H. AUDEN

Kathryn H. Anthony and Barry D. Riccio
309 West Pennsylvania Avenue Urbana, IL 61801 USA
e-mail: kanthony@uiuc.edu or cfbdr@eiu.edu
December 2000

Dear family and friends,

Greetings! Our note this time is briefer than usual. We have spent
the past two years working on our book, *Running for Our Lives: The
Odyssey of Our Battle with Cancer*. It should be out in 2001. If you
would like more information, please let us know. Our book describes
our seven-year saga better than any of our holiday letters, and hopefully
it can help others facing life-threatening illnesses. It has been a cathartic
experience to write.

Suffice it to say that we are both alive and as well as can be expected. Barry had a good winter but a very rough spring. The chemotherapy he had been on for the previous year stopped working, and his cancer began to grow again. It is now in about ten sites, including liver and lung. In May he was hospitalized for emergency surgery on the area around his heart. He rebounded and was taking yet another form of chemotherapy this summer, which unfortunately was not successful. This fall he had radiation to his lung plus a different chemotherapy. He continues to require regular blood transfusions. He is hanging in there.

My year at the university has been incredibly busy. I enjoy my teaching, research, and writing but find my schedule exhausting. Maybe I am just getting older. In any case, I am looking forward to the holiday break as we speak. We finally took care of all our house projects that had piled up since our two years away, and the place looks much better now. We enjoyed reconnecting with our Midwestern friends and colleagues this past year. In May we celebrated our 20th anniversary, a milestone for us. We spent the summer out in San Diego and hope to be back there for the holidays.

Once again, thanks so much to all of you who went out of your way to visit, stay in touch, or offer your good wishes throughout the year. We are grateful for your friendship and look forward to hearing from you. We wish you a terrific holiday season and a happy and healthy 2001!

Love, Kathy and Barry

Kathryn H. Anthony
309 West Pennsylvania Avenue Urbana, IL 61801 USA
e-mail: <u>kanthony@uiuc.edu</u>
January 12, 2001

Re: Barry D. Riccio
Born: November 15, 1954
Died: January 10, 2001

Dear family and friends of Barry:

I regret to inform you that our long medical odyssey is now over. Barry passed away on Wednesday, January 10, 2001, at 8 p.m. in Sharp Memorial Hospital, San Diego, California. He was 46. Since he was first diagnosed with leiomyosarcoma in 1993, he had seven operations, several rounds of chemotherapy, radiation, antiangiogenesis therapy, and about 400 blood transfusions. His quest for treatment included five states and scores of doctors, nurses, and medical staff.

Since early November, Barry had been suffering from a high fever and chills that would not go away. Although he had already become very weak, he was still able to travel out to California for the holidays, where he was able to enjoy the sunshine and warm weather. One of his last walks was on Christmas day, when he, my parents, and I walked around Balboa Island and saw the spectacular holiday displays. He was able to make it a block at a time, stopping to sit on the seawall to catch his breath. Shortly after Christmas, he needed a wheelchair. Eventually he was too weak to take a shower, stand up and take his vitamins, or even bend down to tie his shoes. He was like a car whose engine was slowly running out of steam.

This past Monday he was due to begin a new round of chemo-therapy, a last ditch effort to try to stave off his cancer. But his oxygen level was too low, and instead he was admitted to the hospital. Tests revealed that the cancer in his lungs had roared right through him, and now there was no treatment left. He was on an oxygen mask from Monday afternoon through to the end. Up until the last few hours, he was still able to communicate. Nonetheless, it was very difficult to watch. His mother, my parents, and I were with him. His brother and sister-in-law had just visited this past weekend, along with some of our good friends from the Bay Area. The last piece of food he ate was a piece of belated birthday cake that one of our friends had baked especially for him, along with a tangerine that I had brought from home.

On New Year's Day I asked Barry to reflect on his medical odyssey for the last time. Although it was difficult for him to speak at length, here is some of what he had to say:

> At times Kathy thought I would not be doing well enough to get out to California, but I figured I would do better out there than in the Midwest. And in the beginning, I did. I took more Tylenol, I walked a bit more, I spent time in the sun, and I did not have those intense chills, even though my fever did not go away. But after a week or so after arriving in San Diego, I began finding it hard to breathe, not unlike the experience I had last May. As things got progressively worse, we talked more and more with the doctor and it was finally decided that I should have a thoracentesis, i.e. a draining of the right side of my lung. This procedure was very simple, as it turned out, and not especially painful. But I'm not sure how much it relieved me of my burden. In the beginning I felt better. But by the next morning, taking a shower was a formidable experience. So was just going to the bathroom and taking my vitamins. So we all knew something was severely wrong. On New Year's Eve, just walking two blocks to the Royal Thai restaurant was very, very difficult because I would easily get out of breath. I was usually fine sitting down or lying down. And I did as much of that as possible.
>
> I felt I was no longer the man I once was, and that things had come to a head. 2001, I suspected, would indeed be my last year on earth, even though I would make one last bold attempt to try a new chemotherapy and take my chances…I no longer have much energy to speak of. Indeed I have less than that of my 85-year old mother. And I have become a pitiful shell of my former self. If this is the last year, I guess I can

accept that, since I am very worn down by everything that has happened as of late. I only want to be in some comfort and sleep well as I prepare for the big sleep.

Our immediate families are gathered here in San Diego this weekend. No funeral service will be held, but we will be remembering Barry's life together. Barry's ashes will be scattered in the Pacific Ocean.

I am still in California and will be here a while longer before returning home to the Midwest. Since I am still reeling from all of the above, I prefer no phone calls at this time. It is painful for me to discuss what has happened. However, if you wish to send e-mail messages describing any of your special memories about Barry, I would enjoy collecting them.

In lieu of flowers, memorial donations can be sent to the following:

Barry D. Riccio History Fund, Eastern Illinois University Foundation, Brainard House, 1548 4th Street, Charleston, IL 61920.

Sharp Memorial Hospital Infusion Therapy Center, 8008 Frost Street, Suite 300A, San Diego, CA 92123.

Many thanks for all the support you have shown both of us throughout our medical odyssey.

Love,

Kathy

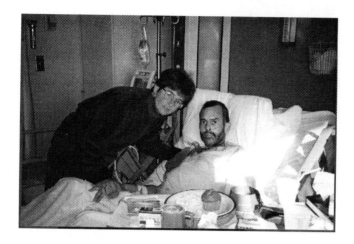

Our final photo together, the last chapter in our medical odyssey. Barry passed away later that evening. San Diego, California, January 2001 (Credit: unknown)

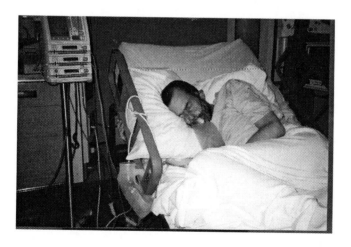

Barry in his final hours. The cancer had spread all over his lungs, and he was on oxygen and morphine until he died. San Diego, California, Janaury 2001 (Credit: Author)

CHRONOLOGY OF
BARRY RICCIO'S CANCER

SUMMARY OF MEDICAL HISTORY

- Born 11/15/54.
- First diagnosed with leiomyosarcoma, cancer of the stomach muscle lining, 9/93 at age 38.
- Metastasized to liver, 10/94 at age 39.
- Recurred in stomach muscle lining and spread to belly cavity, 9/95 at age 40.
- Diagnosed as terminal with approximately 1-3 years left to live, 10/95 at age 40.
- Metastasized to scalp, 1/96; diagnosed 3/97 at age 42.
- Recurred in stomach muscle lining, 7/98 at age 43.
- Metastasized to upper lip, 10/98 at age 43.
- Metastasized to lung, 5/00 at age 45.
- Died 1/10/01 at age 46.

Final medical condition: Extensive cancer in about 12 sites including stomach, liver, abdominal wall, spleen, mesentery, belly cavity, lesser omentum, mediastinum, head, upper lip, near the pericardium, and lung.

Seven operations
1. stomach muscle lining, Carle Hospital, Urbana, IL, 9/93.
   Hospitalized 15 days.
2. liver, MD Anderson Cancer Center, Houston, TX, 12/94.
   Hospitalized 7 days.
3. stomach muscle lining, Carle Hospital, Urbana, IL, 9/95.
   Hospitalized 12 days.
4. greater omentum and belly cavity (photodynamic light therapy)
   Harper Hospital Detroit, MI, 12/95. Hospitalized 7 days.
5. head, Sharp Hospital, San Diego, CA, 4/97. Hospitalized 2
   days.
6. pericardial window (to remove fluid from the cavity around the
   heart) and pleurodesis, Carle Hospital, Urbana, IL, 5/00.
   Hospitalized 8 days.
7. Sphincterotomy (to address a chronic anal fissure) Carle Hospital, Urbana, IL, 5/00. Outpatient surgery. Hospitalized 1 day.

Total: 51 days in hospital

ADDITIONAL OVERNIGHT HOSPITALIZATIONS

GI bleeding, Sharp Hospital, San Diego, CA, 7/98 (6 days).

GI bleeding, Sharp Hospital, San Diego, CA, 8/98 (6 days).

GI bleeding and partial bowel obstruction, Sharp Hospital, San
Diego, CA, 12/98 (7 days).

Transfusions, Sharp Hospital, San Diego, CA, 3/99 (2 days).

Severe back and chest pains, transfusions, Carle Hospital, Urbana,
IL, 11/00 (2 days).

Thoracic cancer, Sharp Hospital, San Diego, CA. 1/01 (3 days).

Total: 26 days in hospital

ADDITIONAL TREATMENTS:

6 rounds of chemotherapy (5FU and Interferon), 1/95 - 7/95.
   Outpatient 48 days.

10 rounds of Vitaxin (a form of antiangiogenesis treatment) @ 6
   weeks each, 2/19/97 through 12/16/98; at the time he discontinued the Vitaxin, Barry survived the longest and had more
   rounds of treatment than any other patient in this phase one
   clinical trial. Outpatient 40 days.

6 weeks of radiation to head, 10/97 - 12/97. Outpatient 30 days.

6-1/2 weeks of radiation to stomach, 9/98 - 11/98. Outpatient 33
   days.

Received approximately 400 units of blood transfusions due to a
   consistently low hemoglobin and GI bleeding, 7/98 – 1/01.
   Hemoglobin level checked every weekday via a blood drawing
   7/98 – 4/00.   Outpatient approximately 110 days;
   Hemoglobin checked twice a week 6/00 – 1/01.
   Outpatient 22 days.

Duodenal stent endoscopically inserted into stomach, 12/98. Barry
   gained 35 pounds. Outpatient 1 day.

Approximately 12 rounds or 950 units of chemotherapy (Cytoxan
   and Adriamycin), 1/99 – 4/00. Outpatient 12 days.

3 rounds of chemotherapy (hi-dose Ifosfamide and Mesna), 6/00 –
   8/00. Outpatient 15 days.

4 rounds of chemotherapy (VePesid or Etoposide in pill form),
   9/00 -11/00.

2-1/2 weeks of radiation to lung, 10/00. Outpatient 13 days.

Right side thoracentesis to remove large right pleural effusion, Sharp Hospital. San Diego, CA, 12/00. Outpatient 1 day.

Total: approximately 338 days as an outpatient

INSTITUTIONS AND DOCTORS INVOLVED IN BARRY'S TREATMENTS

Carle Hospital and Clinic, Urbana, IL, 1993-97, 1999-2000. Dr. Michael Colla, cardiovascular and thoracic surgery; Dr. Michael Day, family practice; Dr. Joel Lans, gastroenterologist; Dr. Patricia Johnson, oncologist; Dr. Ronald E. Sapiente, radiation oncologist; Dr. Lyn Tangen, gastrointestinal surgeon; one additional high risk surgeon. Dr. Patricia Johnson was Barry's primary physician since he was first diagnosed with cancer.

Mayo Clinic, Rochester, MN, 1993. Three physicians, including a specialist in leiomyosarcoma.

MD Anderson Cancer Center, Houston, TX, 1994-95. Dr. Steven A. Curley, Chief, Gastrointestinal Tumor Surgery, specialist in leiomyosarcoma. Dr. Curley served as a medical consultant to Barry throughout his illness.

Harper Hospital, Detroit Medical Center, 1995-96. Dr. David Fromm, Surgeon in Chief.

Sharp Hospital and Clinic/Medical Oncology Associates, San Diego, CA, 1997-2001. Dr. Jurgen Kogler, medical oncology and hematology; Dr. Jeffrey Pressman, gastroenterologist; Dr. Charles Brown, pulmorologist. Dr. Kogler was Barry's primary physician in California.

Sidney Kimmel Cancer Center (SKCC), San Diego, CA, 1997-99. Dr. John Gutheil, Former Director of Clinical Oncology Research.

South Coast Tumor Institute, San Diego, CA, 1997-98. Dr. Ronald S. Scott, Medical Director, radiation oncology and radiologic physics.

UCSD Medical Center, San Diego, CA, 1998. Dr. Kenneth Binmoeller, Director, Gastrointestinal Endoscopy.

MEDICAL RESEARCH CONTACTS

David Cheresh, Ph.D., Professor of Immunology and Vascular Biology, The Scripps Research Institute, La Jolla, CA (inventor of Vitaxin drug along with Peter Brooks).

John Gutheil, M.D., Former Director, Clinical Oncology Research, Sidney Kimmel Cancer Center, La Jolla, CA.

Thomas A. Shiftan, M.D., Medical Director, Oncology, Sharp HealthCare, San Diego, CA; Chairman, Board of Trustees, Sidney Kimmel Cancer Center, La Jolla, CA.

VITAMINS/SUPPLEMENTS BARRY TOOK REGULARLY SINCE INITIAL DIAGNOSIS

Vitamins B, C, E
Echinacea and Goldenseal
Garlic
Selenium

Essiac – approximately 1 year only
Shark Cartilage – approximately 1 year only

PUBLICATIONS ABOUT BARRY RICCIO

"Barry Daniel Riccio. (Nov. 15, 1954-Jan. 15-2001)." *The San Diego Union-Tribune* (January 24, 2001), County Obituaries, p. B-6.

Cook, Anne. "EIU Professor Loses Battle With Cancer." *The News-Gazette* (Champaign-Urbana, IL), (February 6, 2001), p. B-4.

Cook, Anne. "Urbana Man Gets Tumor-Shrinking Drug." *The News-Gazette* (Champaign-Urbana, IL), (May 9, 1998), pp. A-1, A-20.

Crewdson, John. "Test Drug Linked to a Cancer's Remission: It's part of new therapy to limit blood to tumor." *Chicago Tribune* (May 25, 1998), Section 1, p.3.

Gorman, Christine. "The Hope & The Hype: Last week's breathless reports of an imminent cure were, of course, too good to be true. Still, these are exciting times in cancer research." *Time* (May 18, 1998), pp. 38-44.

Kiernan, Vincent. "Scientists Raise Doubts About Widely Publicized Cancer Drugs: They say new therapy may not work in humans, even though Harvard professor's experiments show success in trials with mice." *The Chronicle of Higher Education* 44:36 (May 15, 1998), p. A-20.

"Living with Leiomyosarcoma." *SKCC (Sidney Kimmel Cancer Center) News*, (Fall 1997), p. 8.

Nesmith, Jeff. "Health Watch: Cautious Optimism on Cancer." *The Atlanta Journal-Constitution* (May 5, 1998), p. D-3.

Novarro, Leonard. "The Discoverer: Scripps scientist's work offers big hope for cancer patients." *The San Diego Union-Tribune*, (October 4, 1998), Health Section, p. 7.

Ondash, E'Louise. "Chasing a Cure for Cancer: San Diego-area researchers at work on several promising drugs." *North County Times,* (May 11, 1998), p. D-1.

Shelton, Anita. "Message from the Chair." *History at Eastern, Annual Newsletter of the History Department at Eastern Illinois University,* Charleston, IL (July 2001), pp. 1-2, 9.

SAMPLE PUBLICATIONS BY BARRY RICCIO
(Note: A complete list is available from the author)

BOOKS
Riccio, Barry. *Walter Lippmann: Odyssey of a Liberal.* New Brunswick, NJ: Transaction Publishers, 1993. (paperback edition, 1996) Reviewed in:

- *Journal of American History* (March 1995)
- *Journalism Quarterly* (1994).

Riccio, Barry. *The United States Since 1975.* London, U.K.: Longman Press, part of Longman History of America series (unpublished book manuscript in progress at the time of his death.) Completed essays include: A New Social Contract? A Reagan Revolution. American Family Reconsidered. Blood and Sand: Conflict in the Persian Gulf. Culture Wars. Deficit Politics. Democrats' Despair. Downsizing. Politics of Health. Reagan's Children. Still the Golden Door? Strange Career of Tax Reform. Supply Side. The End of Welfare.

Waldrep, Christopher, Lynne Curry, and Barry D. Riccio, with Terry Barnhart, Dolores Archimbault, John McElligott, Martin Hardeman. *The U.S. Constitution and the Nation: Documents Reader.* NY: Forbes Custom Publishing, 1998. (Collection of primary sources)

ARTICLES

Riccio, Barry D. "Clio from the Right: the Case of Continuity." In Ronald Lora and William H. Longton (ed.), *The American Conservative Press.* Westport: CT: Greenwood Press, 1997.

Riccio, Barry D. "New York Intellectual: The Case of Irving Howe." *Journal of American Culture 19*:3 (Fall 1996), pp. 75-85.

Riccio. Barry D. "Popular Culture and High Culture: Dwight Macdonald, His Critics and the Ideal of Cultural Hierarchy in Modern America." *Journal of American Culture 16:*4 (Winter 1993), pp. 7-18. Received the Carl Bode Award for the best article published in the *Journal of American Culture*, 1993.

Riccio, Barry D. "Richard Nixon Reconsidered: The Conservative as Liberal?" in Leon Friedman and William Levantrosser (eds.). *Watergate and Afterward.* Westport, CT: Greenwood Press, 1992, pp. 279-294.

Riccio, Barry D. "The U.S. Presidency and the Ratings Game.*" The Historian 52*:4 (August 1990), pp. 566-583.

Contributed several biographical sketches in Nancy Weatherly Sharp and James Roger Sharp (eds*.), American Legislative Leaders in the Midwest, 1911-1994.* Westport, CT: Greenwood Press, 1997.

Contributor to D. R. Woolf (ed.) *A Global Encyclopedia of Historical Writing.* NY and London: Garland Publishing Inc., 1998.

CONFERENCE PRESENTATIONS

Riccio, Barry D. "The End of the Republican Era." Mid-America Conference on History." Lawrence, KS, September 18, 1992.

Riccio, Barry D. "Into the Fever Swamps: The Radical Right

Revisited."   Mid-American Conference on History, Springfield, MO, September 15, 1995 (delivered by a colleague while Barry was hospital-ized).

Riccio, Barry D. "New York Intellectual: The Case of Irving Howe." Popular Culture/American Culture Association, Las Vegas, NV, March 28, 1996.

REMEMBER BARRY WHENEVER YOU...

- Drink...Merlot wine...almond sunset, Bengal spice, or red zinger tea
- Line up for food at a buffet
- See his four favorite words in the English language: "All You Can Eat"
- Eat...pasta with rich tomato meat sauce...deep-dish pizza...beef panang (Thai)...samosas (Indian)...Kansas City BBQ sauce...spicy mustards...cinnamon...nutmeg... curry...sweet potatoes...mint meltaway candies...Hershey's kisses...Baskin Robbins' ice cream pies...a second portion...and maybe a third...
- Ask your restaurant server to recite all the ingredients of the meal you are about to order
- Buy a cookbook
- Smell pinon or mesquite in the air
- Sniff a scented candle...favorite flavors: apple, chocolate truffle, cinnamon, mango, spiced pumpkin, tangerine
- Use cedar-scented shoe trees
- Spend an hour or two in a used book store...or in a café reading and greeting the locals
- Stack as many books as possible on your bookshelf until it sags but does not break
- Watch "Crossfire," "Hardball"..."The News Hour with Jim Lehrer"..."This Week"..."Washington Week" on TV
- Read... *The New York Times*... *The New York Review of*

Books...Washington Post Weekly

- Write inside the covers of your books with microscopic text that only you can decipher
- See a play... favorite playwrights: Edward Albee, Sidney Kingsley, David Mamet, Clifford Odets, Eugene O'Neill, Oscar Wilde, Tennessee Williams...favorite themes: courtroom dramas, sibling rivalry
- Watch a classic film... favorite directors: Woody Allen, Alfred Hitchcock, Billy Wilder...favorite actors...Audrey Hepburn, Marlon Brando, James Dean, Cary Grant, James Stewart, Meryl Streep
- Hear Billy Joel's "Piano Man"...Bruce Springsteen's "Born to Run;" soundtracks from "Cinema Paradiso"... "The Godfather"..."Il Postino"..."Life is Beautiful"..."Platoon" ..."Schindler's List;" "Vilkommen" from "Cabaret;" "Route 66"
- Paint something peach
- Keep a messy wallet
- Find scraps of paper, receipts and coins in your pockets
- Can't find your desk beneath all the piles of paper
- Wear out your socks until you get holes in the toes
- See someone...wearing a Greek fisherman's cap...carrying an armload of books...walking at high speed
- Go out for a walk regardless of weather
- Test your vocabulary to find just the right word
- Wish you had a photographic memory...for phone numbers, names, dates, what you were wearing and when
- Look up an old friend
- Consider donating blood
- Don't complain—no matter how bad things may get
- Make the most of each day that finds you in good health
- Feel like giving up—even until the bitter end, he never did

Kathryn H. Anthony is Professor and Chair of the Design
Program Faculty in the School of Architecture at the University of
Illinois at Urbana-Champaign, where she is also an associated faculty
member in the Gender and Women's Studies Program and Department
of Landscape Architecture. She is the author of two books, *Designing
for Diversity: Gender, Race, and Ethnicity in the Architectural Profession*
(University of Illinois Press, 2001) and *Design Juries on Trial: The
Renaissance of the Design Studio* (Van Nostrand Reinhold, 1991), and
scores of scholarly publications. She received the 2003 Collaborative
Achievement Award from the American Institute of Architects (AIA) as
well as the 1992 Creative Achievement Award from the Association of
Collegiate Schools of Architecture. Her work has been cited in *US
News & World Report* and *The Wall Street Journal.*   Her photographs
were published in *Architecture 2002* and *Architecture 1992,* the calendar
of the AIA, and received Honorable Mention in an AIA National
Photography Competition.   Ms. Anthony holds a Bachelors degree in
psychology and a Ph.D. in architecture from the University of California, Berkeley.

In writing *Running for Our Lives,* Ms. Anthony draws upon her
personal diary, extensive interviews with her late husband, Barry Riccio,
and comments from Barry's medical staff. Throughout their medical
odyssey she served as a strong patient advocate, searching for pioneering
research and clinical trials; corresponding with scores of physicians,
medical researchers, family and friends across the country; and accompanying Barry on hundreds of medical appointments. She used 13 years
of accumulated sick leave to travel with Barry for medical treatment.

Barry D. Riccio was Associate Professor of History at Eastern
Illinois University in Charleston, Illinois. He also taught at the Univer-
sity of California at Berkeley; the University of Illinois at Urbana-
Champaign; Knox College; Illinois Wesleyan University; California
State Polytechnic University, Pomona; and at four community colleges
in Illinois and California. He was the author of *Walter Lippmann:
Odyssey of A Liberal,* (Transaction Publishers, 1993) and numerous
scholarly publications. A specialist in 20th century American social

thought and Presidential politics, he received the 1994 Carl Bode Award from the American Culture Association. He appeared on CSPAN on the meaning of Richard Nixon's presidency and on WILL National Public Radio. Mr. Riccio was also a playwright; his play, "The Review," was performed at the Charleston Alley Theatre in Charleston, Illinois in 1997. Friends also knew him as a highly accomplished chef. Mr. Riccio held a Ph.D. in history from the University of California at Berkeley and a Masters in history and a Bachelors degree in political science, both from the University of Illinois at Chicago.

For over seven years, Mr. Riccio battled leiomyosarcoma, cancer of the stomach muscle lining, which spread to his liver, greater omentum, belly cavity, abdomen wall, mesentery, spleen, head, lip, and lung. In 1998 he was catapulted into the role of spokesperson for the anti-angiogenesis movement, featured on ABC Evening News with Peter Jennings and highlighted in the "In Their Own Words" segment of NBC Nightly News with Tom Brokaw. He was interviewed by *Time*, *The Atlanta Journal-Constitution*, *The Chicago Tribune*, *The Los Angeles Times*, and *The Chronicle of Higher Education*. He also received coverage in *The News Gazette* (Champaign-Urbana, Illinois), *North County Times* (San Diego County), and on San Diego's local television news. He died in San Diego, California in 2001 at age 46.

The authors met as graduate students at International House, University of California, Berkeley. They were married for 20 years.